ALSO BY DONNA HOHMANN EWY AND RODGER FRANK EWY:

Preparation for Childbirth

Preparation for Breastfeeding

The Cycle of Life
Guide to a Healthy Pregnancy
Guide to Parenting: You and Your Newborn

Hoberman/May

Niswander Obstetrics

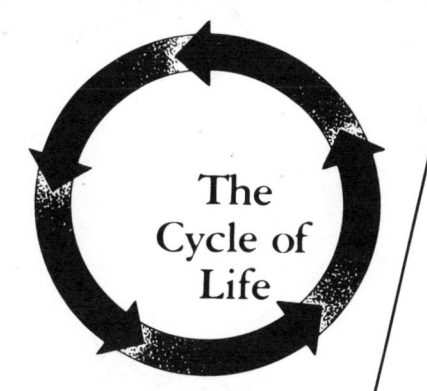

The Cycle of Life

Guide to
FAMILY–CENTERED CHILDBIRTH

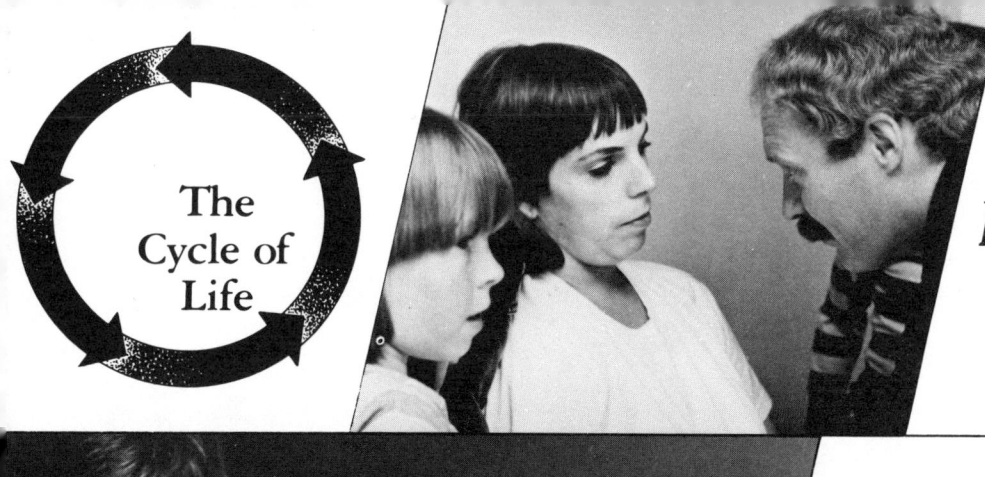

The Cycle of Life

Donna and Rodger Ewy

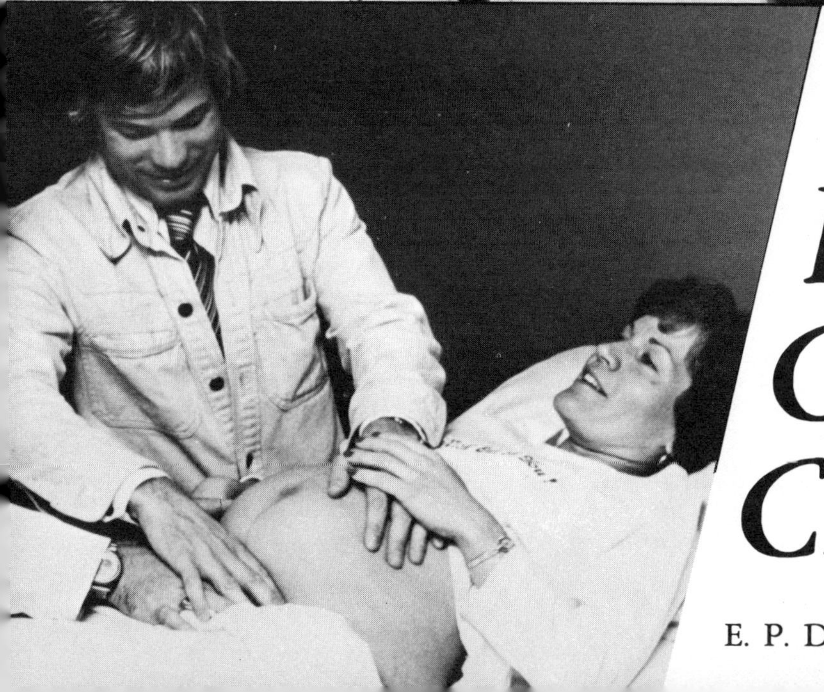

Guide to
FAMILY–CENTERED CHILDBIRTH

E. P. DUTTON / NEW YORK

Copyright © 1981 by Donna and Rodger Ewy / All rights reserved. Printed in the U.S.A. / No part of this publication may be reproduced or transmitted in any form or by any means, electronic or mechanical, including photocopy, recording or any information storage and retrieval system now known or to be invented, without permission in writing from the publisher, except by a reviewer who wishes to quote brief passages in connection with a review written for inclusion in a magazine, newspaper or broadcast / Published in the United States by E. P. Dutton, Inc., 2 Park Avenue, New York, N.Y. 10016 / Library of Congress Cataloging in Publication Data / Ewy, Donna / Guide to family-centered childbirth / (Their The cycle of life) / Bibliography: p. 173 / 1. Childbirth. 2. Labor (Obstetrics) I. Ewy, Rodger, joint author. II. Title. III. Series: Cycle of life. [DNLM: 1. Family—Popular works. 2. Labor—Popular works. WQ 150 E95ca] RG651.E9 1981   618.4   80-26481 / ISBN: 0-525-93183-X / Published simultaneously in Canada by Clarke, Irwin & Company Limited, Toronto and Vancouver / 10 9 8 7 6 5 4 3 2 1 / First Edition

*To our children
and to all the dedicated pioneers
who made
family-centered childbirth
a reality*

A Baby's Ten Commandments to Parents During Childbirth

Dear Parent:

Many things happen during your labor and my delivery that will affect me for the rest of my life. Your attitude and choices during this most vulnerable time are crucial to my physical and emotional development.

1. Please consider my birth as a normal, healthy process in which both of you, my mother and my father, will be active participants.
2. Please select a doctor or medical caregiver (birthing attendant) who will be concerned not only with the physical, but with the emotional health of our family.
3. Please choose a birth place which ensures minimal use of intervention techniques for low-risk births, while at the same time offering the best obstetrical techniques for high-risk births should they be needed.
4. Since there is no medication which does not have some effect on me both during and immediately following birth, please take as little medication as possible if we are to have a normal and uncomplicated labor and delivery.
5. Since there is no medical intervention or obstetrical technique that does not carry with it some risks, please choose a medical birthing attendant whose philosophy ensures minimum intervention, used only when medically indicated.
6. Please choose a birthing attendant and a birthing site which allows all of us

(mother, father, and baby) the quiet, calm, gentleness, and dignity which befits the birth of our family.

7. If at all possible, please choose to be awake during my birth, for it will be one of the most exciting and creative events of all our lives.
8. Please let your doctor and hospital know that you wish to have early and extended contact with me and that it is important that you be allowed to hold me in your arms, explore me and love me immediately following birth.
9. Please pick a birthing place which will give you the vital information and support you will need on feeding, caring for, and nurturing me.
10. Though I am a combination of both of you, I am a complete and unique individual with my own unique personality. Take time to get to know me. I am yours to explore, hold, kiss, touch, fondle and love. I am yours for the rest of your lives.

Thank you,
Your loving child

Contents

Acknowledgments *xiii*
Introduction *xv*
1. Family-centered Childbirth *1*
2. Passageway, Passenger, and Powers *7*
3. The Birth Process *23*
4. Alleviating Pain in Childbirth *29*
5. Controlled Relaxation and Concentration *33*
6. Controlled Breathing *47*
7. Expulsion Techniques *59*
8. Comforting Techniques *65*
9. Birth *73*
10. Family-centered Alternatives *111*
11. Possible Problems in Labor and Birth *123*
12. Cesarean Childbirth *127*
13. Medical Intervention and Anesthetics *145*
14. Being Prepared for All Eventualities *159*
    Glossary *165*
    Further Reading *173*

Acknowledgments

We would like especially to thank the following people who shared their time, energy, and information with us:

First, our parents who gave us our first important lessons in parenting. Next, our children Marguerite, Suzanne, Rodger, and Leon, who have unceasingly tested our own parenting techniques and given us invaluable experiences.

Our special appreciation goes to the many pregnant parents who have shared their experiences and families with us: Ann and Sam Baron, Anne and K. L. Berry, Minnie Cordova, Anita and Andre DePriest, Lynn and Ken Ewall, Tommy and Ron Farina, Gail and Dave Hall, Kathy and Mike Hinojos, Mike and Cecile Lederhos, Ted and Stacey Levin, Linda Loeb, Sherry Mulloy, Jeannie Paxton, Jim and Donnette Raabe, Roberta and Bob Scaer, Robyn and Rick Sears, Peggy Smith, Dennis Surina, Kay Wilson, and Cindy Yeoman.

We are especially grateful for the information and critiques shared so generously by our professional consultants: Kathy Bernau, R.N., M.S., Coordinator of Patient Education, Rose Medical Center, Denver; Watson Bowes, Jr., M.D., Chairman, Department of Obstetrics / Gynecology, University of Colorado School of Medicine, Denver; T. Berry Brazelton, M.D., Chief, Child Development Unit, The Children's Hospital Medical Center, and Associate Professor of Pediatrics, Harvard Medical School, Cambridge; Joseph Butterfield, M.D., Chairman, Department of Perinatology, Children's Hospital, Denver; William Clewell, M.D., Assistant Professor of Obstetrics / Gynecology, University of Colorado School of Medicine, Denver; Harvey M. Cohen, M.D., Department of Obstetrics / Gynecology St. Anthony's Hospital, Denver; Robert Emde, M.D., Professor of Psychiatry, University of Colorado School of Medicine, Denver; Bob Harmon, M.D., Assistant Professor of Child Psychiatry, University of Colorado School of Medicine, Denver; Trudy Hutchinson, Registered Dietician, Nutrition Service, University of Colorado Medical Center, Denver; Betty Jennings, Certified Nurse Midwife/Practitioner, Obstetrics Clinic, University of Colorado Medical Center, Denver; William Kimberling, Ph.D., Assistant Professor of Genetics, Department of Pediatrics, University of Colorado School of Medicine, Denver; Marshall H. Klaus, M.D., Professor of Pediatrics, Case Western Reserve University, Cleveland; Mary Krugman, R.N., M.S., Coordinator of Parent Education, Rose Medical Center, Denver; Richard Krugman, M.D., Associate Professor of Pediatrics, Codirector of Child Health Associate Program, University of Colorado School of Medicine, Denver; Heidi Lynch, R.P.T., C.C.E., American Society for Psychoprophylaxis in Obstetrics Trainer, Boulder; Patricia O'Connor, R.N., C.C.E., Assistant Coordinator, Nurses Association of the American College of Obstetricians and Gynecologists, Vice Chairman, American Society for Psychoprophylaxis in Childbirth, Denver; Doug Pugh, M.D., Clinical Neonatology Fellow, Division of Perinatal Medicine, University of Colorado Medical Center, Denver; Reva Rubin, Professor, Department of Maternity Nursing, University of Pittsburgh; Pamela Shrock, R.P.T., M.P.M., Clinical Nurse Consultant, Chicago; Vicki Walton, Manager, The Birthplace, Seattle; Paul Wexler, M.D., Chairman, Dept. of Obstetrics / Gynecology, Rose Medical Center, Denver and Assistant Clinical Professor, University of Colorado School of Medicine, Denver; and Marelynn W. Zipser, Ph.D., Nutritionist.

Paula Lehr and Rebecca Metcalfe have our great appreciation for the many hours they spent at the typewriter.

To our editors, Sally Crowley, Patti Hodgins, Marian Skedgell, Karen Braziller, and Amelie Littell, our thanks for their important contributions.

Finally, we would like to thank our good friend Warren Rovetch, who had the vision to see in print the books *The Cycle of Life: Guide to a Healthy Pregnancy, Guide to Family-centered Childbirth,* and *Guide to Parenting: You and Your Newborn.*

Introduction

The field of childbirth has changed profoundly in the past twenty years. Where patients once submitted themselves unquestioningly to scientific and medical authority, now pregnant parents play an active and responsible role in one of the most creative acts of their lives: the birth of their family. They and their babies are reaping the benefits of high-technology obstetrics along with the humanistic benefits of family-centered childbirth.

This book, *Guide to Family-centered Childbirth,* is designed not only to give you information about what is happening to you and what to expect, but, most important of all, to give you ways of dealing with and remaining in control of your experience in childbirth.

Childbirth is one of life's turning points. It may be one of the first major crises that you, as a couple, face together. Getting information, developing techniques, and seeking a support system are all positive and constructive ways to face any crisis. Childbirth without preparation may be frightening and threatening, whereas childbirth with preparation can be an experience in which you grow and flourish. How you deal with this event very often sets up a pattern that your family will follow in facing other turning points that are sure to appear in your life.

Guide to Family-centered Childbirth gives you, the pregnant parent, information about the mechanics of labor and delivery and what is happening to your body. It gives you, the laboring mother, the techniques you will need to meet the growing intensity of the uterine contractions during labor and delivery. And finally, it gives you, the coaching partner, the information and techniques you will need to give encouragement, instruction, and comfort to the laboring mother. It provides a step-by-step description of both your roles as you progress from early labor through the birth itself.

There is no one "storybook" labor or delivery. Everyone's experience with childbirth is individual, and so will yours be. Although no one can determine the type of labor you will have, this book will prepare you for almost any experience that might confront you, including complications and cesarean birth, and all in a family-centered context.

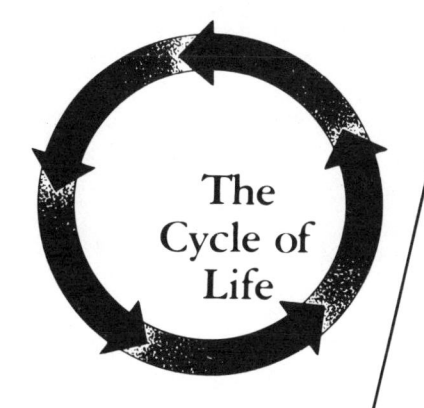

The Cycle of Life

Guide to
FAMILY–CENTERED CHILDBIRTH

1.

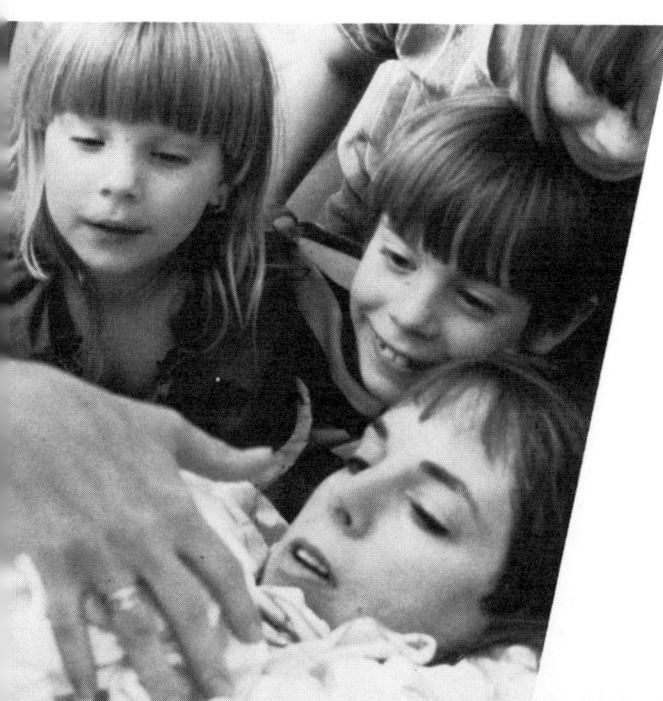

Family-centered Childbirth

Throughout much of history, pregnancy and childbirth posed great risks; many women and babies died during childbirth. With the advent of anesthesia and hospital birth, obstetrical intervention became part of the scene. Knowledge and support were taken from the family as a unit. The mother in labor was admitted to the hospital, placed in a sterile, unfamiliar room, and given a shave, an enema, and medication. She labored alone while the father paced helplessly in the "father's waiting room." When the time for birth was near, the mother was taken to the delivery room and laid on her back on a table, her legs strapped into position in metal stirrups and her arms strapped at her sides. Anesthetized and unable to participate in the birth, the mother had her baby "delivered" to her. The father, waiting anxiously, was told of the birth of his child by a relative stranger. The mother, baby, and father were then separated for an extended period. For the first time in a long recorded history of humankind, the majority of young people lost their role as partners in the important sequence of birth and parenting.

Meanwhile, over the years, there has been a steady decline of mother and baby mortality rates. This decline has been due not only to advances in high-risk obstetrical technology and the availability of antibiotics, but also to parents' increased knowledge of hygiene, nutrition, family planning, and the willingness of pregnant parents to assume their responsibilities in a healthy pregnancy and childbirth. However, the traditional hospital scene persisted. "There must be another way" was a cry that echoed from parents to the caring doctors and nurses who accompanied them on their voyage to becoming a family. Thus was born a movement that slowly evolved into family-centered childbirth.

NATURAL CHILDBIRTH

In the 1930s, Dr. Grantly Dick-Read, author of *Natural Childbirth,* was the first to suggest that childbirth need not be painful, and that the pain of labor and delivery came from cultural expectations rather than from physiological causes. He theorized the "fear-tension-pain" syndrome: Fear produces tension in the muscles, which in turn results in feelings of pain. He suggested that if a woman has no fear, she can relax and experience no pain. Although Grantly Dick-Read made important contributions, the method was criticized for inducing feelings of guilt or failure if a woman did indeed experience pain during childbirth.

THE LAMAZE METHOD OF CHILDBIRTH (PSYCHOPROPHYLAXIS)

Several decades later, a group of Russian scientists became interested in analyzing the components of pain and in preventing it by changing the individual's perceptions. Psychoprophylaxis is based on the works of Pavlov, who first understood that perception of stimuli takes place in the brain. For every stimulus there is a response that can be conditioned (learned) by repetition or practice.

Psychoprophylaxis means "mind-prevention," or prevention of pain through conditioning of the brain. When a person receives any painful stimulus (be it a pinprick, a burn, or the contractions of the uterus during childbirth), a message is sent through the nerves to the brain. There it is interpreted and some response chosen. The Pavlovians theorized that if a person is educated to perceive the painful stimulus as a positive force, and conditioned or trained to respond to it in a positive way, the pain can be eliminated or alleviated. It was also theorized that the brain can only process a certain amount of information at one time, and that if it receives a large number of stimuli or impulses, the individual's perception of the painful stimulus will be diminished or decreased.

Russian obstetricians who were interested in psychoprophylaxis brought these theories into obstetrics. In 1954 Velvosky presented psychoprophylaxis as a method by which childbirth could become a positive conditioned process. A woman may be conditioned by society to interpret her contractions as a painful sensation to which a common response would be to scream or become tense. On the other hand, the same woman can be educated to interpret her contractions as a mechanism that gives birth to her child, and she can be conditioned to respond with a variety of techniques that alleviate or eliminate painful sensation in childbirth. Techniques such as conscious relaxation and deep breathing were introduced to diminish perception of the intensity of the uterine contractions. Thus, psychoprophylaxis was based on

1. education to decondition a woman's expectation of pain
2. conditioning to teach her to respond with relaxation and deep breathing

Psychoprophylaxis made a significant contribution to prepared childbirth as we know it today.

When psychoprophylaxis was introduced to the Western obstetrical world in 1951, a French obstetrician, Fernand Lamaze, became interested in the method and brought it to his hospital in Paris. He modified the breathing techniques to include rapid and panting breathing, and also introduced the use of controlled neuromuscular relaxation and a type of massage called effleurage. Renaming psychoprophylaxis "accouchement sans douleur" or "childbirth without pain," Lamaze emphasized avoiding pain rather than coping with painful stimuli.

OTHER DISCOVERIES

We are only now beginning to realize the significance of the events that surround the birth process. Recent research emphasizes the importance of the participation of the whole family immediately after birth when bonding, the development of feelings of attachment, takes place. Doctors Marshall Klaus and John Kennell, pioneer neonatologists, traced the development of the attachment process from pregnancy through the first hours of birth and the events and procedures that influence the early development of the family. They identified those factors that enhanced or inhibited the attachment processes. Common procedures, such as separating mother and baby immediately following birth, were shown to inhibit the attachment process. Klaus and Kennell found that allowing the family this special time together fostered parent-child bonding.

Reva Rubin and others have described the emotional aspects of pregnancy and childbirth. Stress and high anxiety levels were correlated with high risks in pregnancy and childbirth.

Dr. T. Berry Brazelton had given us important information on the capabilities of the newborn and his ability to affect the interaction between himself and his parents. Detailed studies have shown that a newborn baby moves in rhythm to his mother's voice in the first minutes and hours of life. The baby's appearance and his sensory and motor reactions elicit responses from the mother and provide the parents feedback that is essential in the process of attachment.

FAMILY-CENTERED CHILDBIRTH TODAY

Today, family-centered childbirth means a humanized integrated approach in which the best methods have been individualized to meet the varied needs of all parents. Family-centered childbirth gives parents responsibility, involvement, choice, and control in the birth of their baby. It uses present-day knowledge of high-risk obstetrics, neonatology, and infant development along with the concepts of humanized birth and the importance of parent-infant attachment. Family-centered maternity care offers an atmosphere, facilities, and a supporting staff that foster the development of warm and loving feelings between the newborn and the family.

Benefits of Preparation

There has been a great deal of research on the physiological and psychological effects of childbirth preparation in mothers, fathers, and babies. Some studies report that training results in decreased perception of pain by the mother. Increased cooperativeness on the part of the mother during labor, a decreased incidence of postpartum depression and a more positive attitude regarding future pregnancy have also been documented. Other studies state that training results in benefits from an obstetrical point of view, including reduced use of analgesic and anesthetic medication; less blood loss; a decrease in the incidence of significant obstetrical interventions, including forceps deliveries, episiotomies, and cesarean section; and a significant decrease in the length of labor. Still other research describes benefits to the child, including increased oxygenation of fetal blood, more rapid initiation of breathing following expulsion, a decreased incidence of the necessity for resuscitation, better adjustment to the nursery, and a decrease in the rate of neonatal mortality and illness.

Taken as a whole, these studies suggest that childbirth preparation carries a number of physical and psychological benefits for mother, child, and family. However, the most important research finding is that childbirth preparation is an important preventive mental health measure. No matter how long or hard the labor, trained mothers feel better about themselves, their babies, and their husbands. Prepared parents view childbirth as a positive experience. They perceive themselves as being in control of their labor and delivery, and their self-esteem is enhanced with the birth of their child.

A Family-centered Support System

The components of a good birthing situation for a low-risk mother are:

1. Both parents prepared to be active participants in the birth of their child.
2. A participating and supporting medical team.
3. Options that offer parents freedom and flexibility.
4. Concern for the comfort of the mother during labor and delivery.
5. Minimal medical and obstetrical intervention.
6. No separation from baby for either parent during the sensitive period immediately following birth.

Since the choice of doctor (or birthing attendant), hospital (or birthing site), and childbirth preparation class are some of the most important choices of your life, you must give great care to the task. If you do not ask for a family-centered childbirth experience you will probably be given the traditional routine treatment throughout your labor, delivery, and postpartum. Be specific about your wish for a family-centered childbirth and make sure your wish is understood *before* the birth of your child. (For guidelines to help you select a family-centered birthing attendant, birthing site, and childbirth class, see *The Cycle of Life: Guide to a Healthy Pregnancy*.)

2.

Passageway, Passenger, and Powers

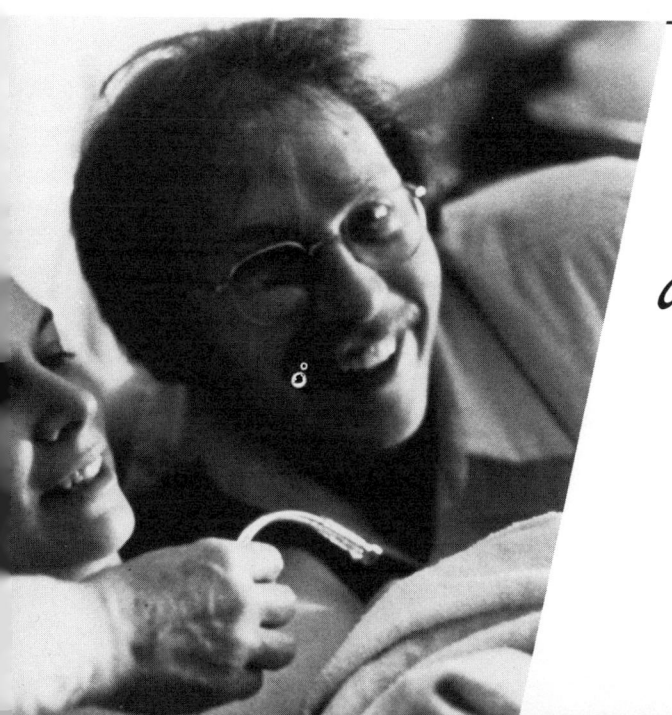

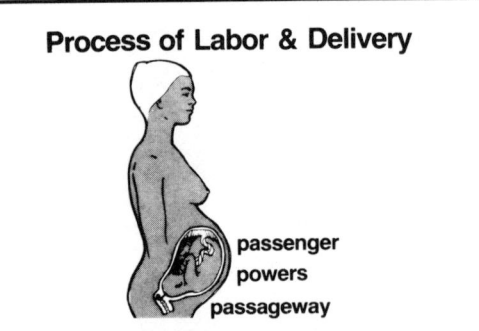

One of the most important aspects of prepared childbirth is being knowledgeable about the processes of labor and delivery. Being informed will help you know what is happening, why it is happening, and how you can cope with the normal and natural phenomena that are taking place during the birth of your baby.

The three basic elements in the birthing process are: the mother's reproductive system and the passageway through which the baby normally travels; the size and position of the baby; and the powers that help expel the baby at birth. Normal labor and delivery depend on the adequate size and shape of your pelvis (the passageway); the size, position, and presentation of your baby (the passenger); and the efficiency and adequacy of your uterine contractions (the power).

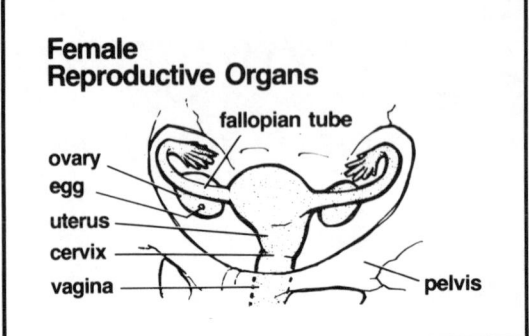

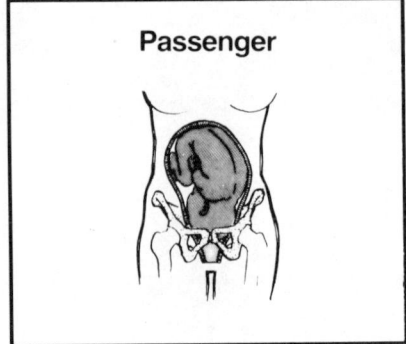

THE PASSAGEWAY

Uterus

The uterus is a hollow muscular organ located in the pelvis above the pubic bone. It resembles a small pear in size and shape and is about three inches long and two inches wide at the top. The outside of the uterus has many elastic fibers meshed with powerful muscle fibers, allowing it to expand for the growing fetus and for the delivery of the baby. The inside of your uterus is a narrow, triangle-shaped cavity covered by a red, velvety lining called the endometrium, which provides nutrients to the fertilized egg.

Your uterus is divided into two parts: the body and the cervix. The body, the main part of your uterus, houses and protects your baby. The top of the uterus is called the fundus. The cervix is the opening between the body of the uterus and the vagina, or birth canal.

The muscles of your uterus are arranged in an outer, a middle, and an inner layer. The outer layer arches over the top of your uterus and extends down toward your pubic bone. The internal layer is made up of fibers that surround the openings of the fallopian tubes and the cervix. The middle layer is a network of interlacing muscle fibers, running in all directions, each forming a figure eight, and overlapping one another in shinglelike arrangements.

These muscle layers expand and grow tremendously to accommodate the growth of your baby. Your uterus will grow from 2½ ounces to 2½ pounds, and its capacity will increase over 500 times during pregnancy.

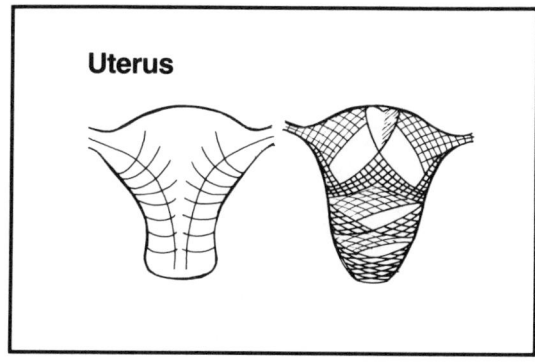

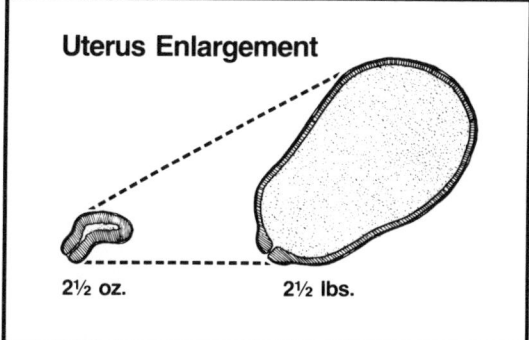

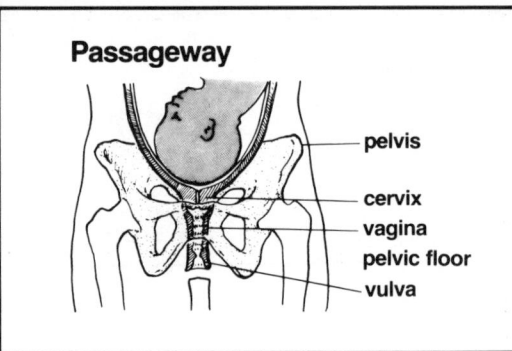

Cervix

The cervix, which makes up the passageway from your uterus to the birth canal, is tubular and measures about one inch from the internal end that opens from the uterus to the external part that opens into the vagina. The space between the two openings is filled with a mucous plug that protects the uterus from external infection. The early contractions of labor loosen the membranes and set free the plug. The cervix is firm and its passageway is so narrow that nothing larger than the lead of a pencil could pass through it easily. Under the strong pressure of childbirth, however, its fibrous material effaces (or thins out) and finally opens to the size of your baby's head.

Vagina

The vagina is a protected passageway for the sperm. It is also your organ of intercourse, the passageway for menstrual flow, and the route for your baby to descend from the uterus to the outside world. It is located behind the bladder and in front of the rectum at an angle in line with the cervix. Ingeniously designed to expand to the size of your baby's head and body, the vagina is from three to five inches long, and its walls are arranged in thick expandable folds. These elastic folds allow the vagina to open to many times its original size for the delivery of your baby.

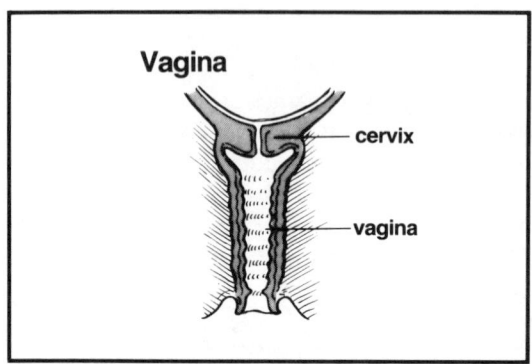

Pelvic Floor

A band of interlacing muscles called the pelvic floor covers the base of your pelvis. These muscles support the internal organs from below and contain the openings that lead from the inner organs to the outside. There are three openings: the urethra, which leads from the bladder; the vagina, which leads from the uterus; and the anus, which leads from the rectum. During childbirth, not only will the opening to the vagina stretch, but the area between the anus and the vagina, which is called the perineum, will stretch as well. As your baby passes through the pelvic floor, the muscles are displaced to make room for him.

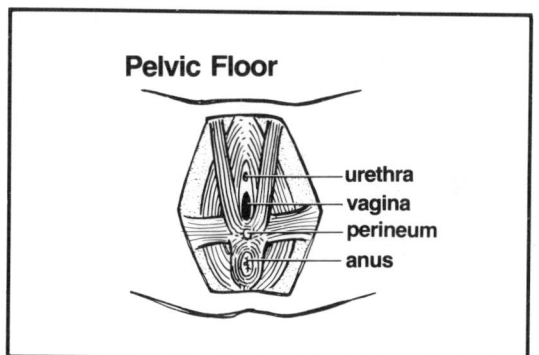

Vulva

The last passage your baby has to make before he emerges into the world is through the external opening of the vagina, which stretches to accommodate his head. Starting from the top, the most visible part of the vulva is the mons veneris or pubis, which covers the pubic bone and serves as a protection for the inner organs. Below is a set of protective folds called the labia majora (or outer lips), which cover and protect the external opening. Inside the large lips are two smaller and thinner folds of more sensitive skin called the labia minora (or inner lips), which end below the entrance to the vagina. Where the upper folds of the lips come together, there is the small and sensitive organ called the clitoris.

Pelvis

Your pelvis is the bony structure that surrounds your baby during pregnancy. It is made up of four bones: the two hipbones; the sacrum, the base of your backbone; and the

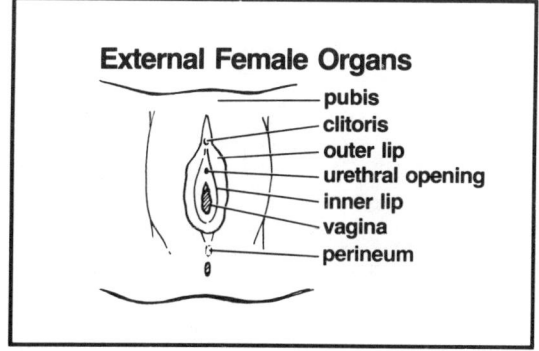

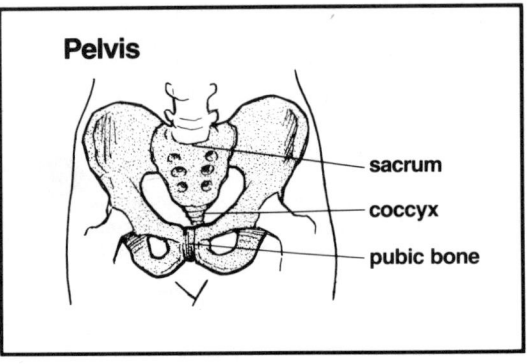

coccyx or tailbone. These bones are joined by cartilage and ligaments that are movable and can expand slightly, giving your pelvis the capacity to widen during pregnancy and birth. In the front, the two hipbones meet each other to form the first joint at the pubic bone. The hipbones join in back at the sacrum and form the second and third joints. And finally, the sacrum and coccyx unite to form the fourth joint.

It may help you to think of your pelvis as a basin which can be viewed three ways. The first view looks at the front of the basin, the second looks at the basin from the side, and the third view looks through the brim to the bottom. The boundaries of your pelvis are important in checking for complications in labor and delivery. If you look down at the pelvis as you would look down on a bowl, you would see the passageway has an inlet at the top and an outlet at the bottom. The three measurements that determine whether your baby's head and body can pass easily through your pelvis are the diameters of (1) the inlet, (2) the outlet, and (3) the passageway between.

INLET

The inlet is formed by your pubic arch in front, by your sacrum in the rear, and by the inner sides of your pelvis at the brim. At the bottom, the outlet is formed by your pubic bone, the coccyx, and two bones called the ischial spines. These are very important landmarks during birth.

An instrument called the pelvimeter may be used to give an approximate measure of the pelvic inlet, which your baby enters early in the birth process. An inlet that measures greater than 13.5 centimeters (cm.) is of adequate size for childbirth. The shape of the normal inlet is oval, with its greater measurement from hip to hip.

OUTLET

Your baby exits from your pelvis at the pelvic outlet. A diameter greater than 11 cm. is considered normal for the average delivery. An internal measurement can be taken by an

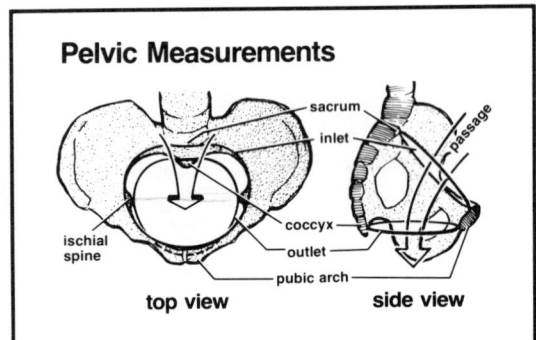

examiner who gently inserts two fingers into your vagina. By feeling the side walls of your pelvis, he can estimate the distance between your ischial spines. He may also measure the distance externally.

The outlet also has an oval shape, but unlike the oval inlet, its greater measurement is from front to back. So, the baby's maneuvering down the passageway is much like putting a foot into a boot where the upper part is wider from side to side and the lower part is wider from front to back.

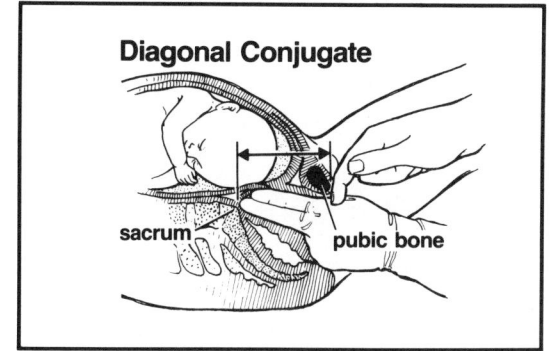

DIAGONAL CONJUGATE

The area of the passageway where your baby has to maneuver this change is called the diagonal conjugate. The measurement of this area is probably the most critical in determining your labor. By feeling the height of your pubic bone, the shape of your pubic arch, the mobility of your tail bone, and the angle of your sacrum, the diagonal conjugate is assessed. If the measurement from your sacrum to the lowest part of your pubic bone is greater than 11.5 cm., your diagonal conjugate is assumed to be adequate for your baby to pass through.

SIZE AND SHAPE

Slight irregularities in the structure of your pelvis may delay the progress of labor, while great irregularities may make delivery by the vaginal passage impossible. There is no perfect pelvis, and no two are the same. Differences are caused by heredity, disease, injury, and nutrition. There are four general types of pelvis: gynecoid, elongated, wedge, and flat.

Gynecoid (normal). About half of all women have the gynecoid or normal type of pelvis. The brim of this type of pelvis is oval, with the widest measurement across the hips.

Elongated (anthropoid). The elongated pelvis is present in about 25 percent of all women. It is the same shape as the gynecoid pelvis, but the oval is turned sideways, so that the widest part is from front to back. Both pelvic types usually result in uncomplicated deliveries.

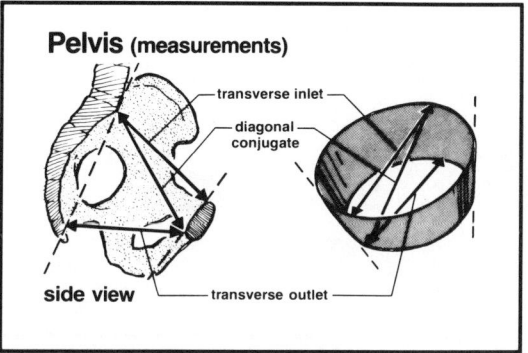

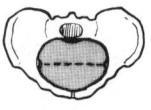 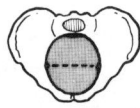

Pelvis (types): gynecoid, anthropoid

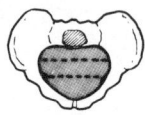 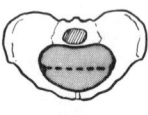

Pelvis (types): android, flat

Wedge (android). About 20 percent of all women have a wedge pelvis. The inlet is a heart-shaped triangle with the widest dimension near the sacrum. This shortens the available diameter and the progress of the baby's head through the pelvis causes increasing problems the further it descends.

Flat. Only five percent of all women are flat pelvic types. The delivery of a baby's head through this pelvis is difficult at the brim, but is easier with further descent.

PASSENGER

The type of childbirth you may experience is affected not only by the adequacy of your passageway; just as important is the passenger himself. Your baby is an active participant in the drama of birth. He has made the miraculous journey from a single cell to a complex individual with a unique physical, emotional, and intellectual potential.

Inner World

Your baby has specialized equipment to use while he lives inside you. He has his own space capsule, the amniotic sac; has his own lifeline, the umbilical cord; and the placenta is his space pack.

PLACENTA

The placenta is one of the most complex organs of the human body. Your baby will use it only as long as he lives inside you; through it, he gathers nutrients and oxygen from your body and passes wastes back out to it. The placenta is a pancake-shaped organ about the size of a salad plate by the time your baby is born. Filled with a network of blood vessels, it performs the many tasks of the kidneys, intestines, liver, endocrine glands, and lungs of an adult. The placenta is also called the "afterbirth," since it is expelled after the baby is born.

UMBILICAL CORD

The umbilical cord is your baby's lifeline. One end of it connects with the placenta; the other leads into your baby's belly at the point that will become his navel. A bright bluish-green tube about twenty inches in length, the umbilical cord is filled with a substance called Wharton's jelly that makes it soft and thick. It loops in a spiral and is long enough to allow your baby to move freely. The cord brings fresh blood from the placenta and returns your baby's waste products. The blood flows under pressure through the cord so that it is always firm, like a garden hose filled with water.

AMNIOTIC SAC

Your baby's space capsule is a sac containing the environment he needs for survival. The fluid-filled space surrounding the baby is called the amniotic cavity, or the "bag of waters." This space has a smooth, slippery lining, the amniotic membrane.

The amniotic fluid that fills the sac is an amber-colored liquid. The fluid keeps your baby at an even temperature, protects him from outside injury, provides a medium in which he can move easily, and lubricates the skin. Through the amniotic membrane, about a third of this fluid is replaced every hour with water from the mother's blood plasma. The amount of fluid present in the cavity decreases as your baby grows larger. At the time of delivery, the cavity contains from one to two pints of fluid. Your baby will live in fluid until his birth. Thus, he never breathes air into his lungs until after he is born. Until then, he gets oxygen from your blood through the placenta.

Size, Position, and Movements

Your baby's size and position help or hinder him as he maneuvers from your uterus through your pelvis and the birth canal to his first breath of life. Your doctor can assess some of these factors when he or she examines you. By outlining the buttocks, back, and head of your baby, the doctor can determine his position in your uterus and the part of his body that may first present itself during the birth.

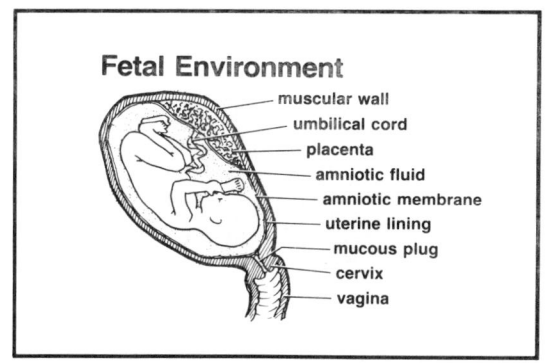

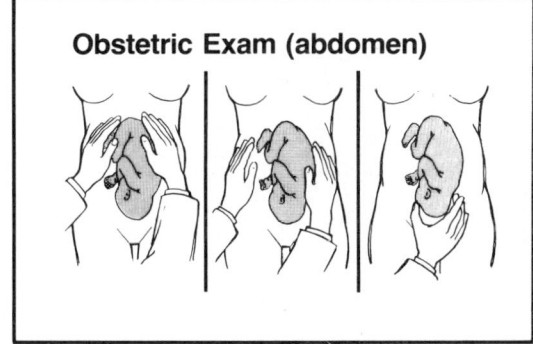

15

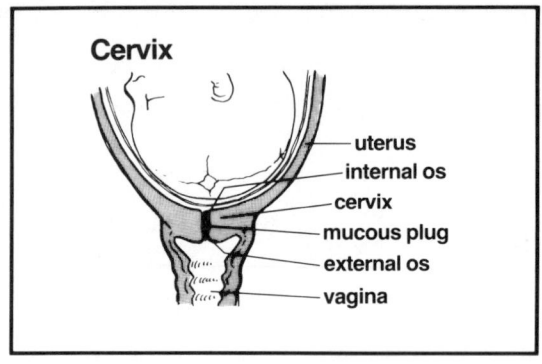

SIZE AND SHAPE OF BABY'S SKULL

The part of your baby that occupies the lower part of your uterus will be the first part to emerge. The baby's head is the most effective wedge on the cervix. When the head of your baby points down into your pelvis, it is said to be a cephalic or vertex presentation. This is the normal way of presenting.

The part of your baby that most influences labor and delivery is his skull. The fetal skull and the female pelvis are made for one another, like a hand fitting into a glove. If the baby's head can pass through your pelvis safely, the rest of his body can be delivered with no trouble. Usually, the smallest part of the back of the head, the occiput, presents itself first.

Just as the inlet and outlet of your pelvis are oval-shaped, so is the shape of your baby's head. The longest diameter of the oval is from front to back, and averages 11.75 cm., the same dimension as the average mother's pelvis. Your baby's skull is made up of eight bones that are not knit tightly together at the time of birth but are separated by membranes called sutures. The intersections of these sutures are called fontanels, or soft spots. There are two fontanels: a large, diamond-shaped one in front, and a small, triangular one in back. By feeling them, an examiner can determine the position of your baby's

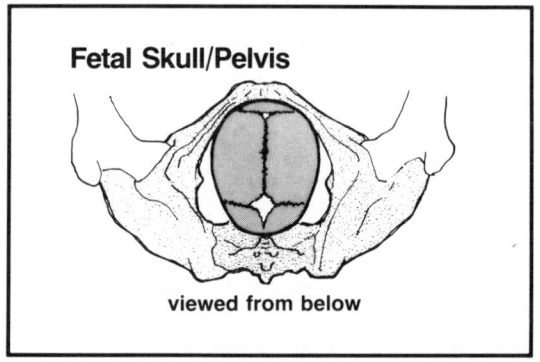

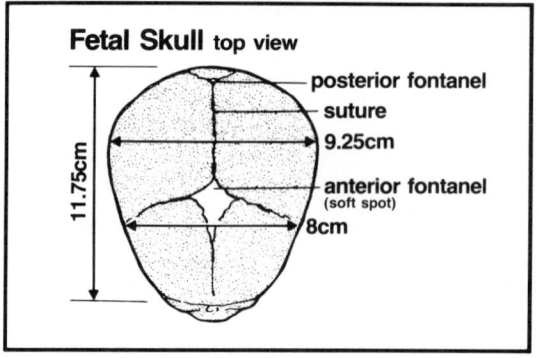

head. The soft spots allow the bones to overlap during labor and reduce the size of your baby's head during his passage through the pelvis.

LIE

For a normal vaginal birth, the direction your baby is lying in relation to your spine is of the utmost importance. This is called the lie. It is considered normal when your baby's spine is parallel with your spine. If your baby is lying across your pelvis, a vaginal birth is impossible, and unless this position changes, a cesarean section will have to be performed.

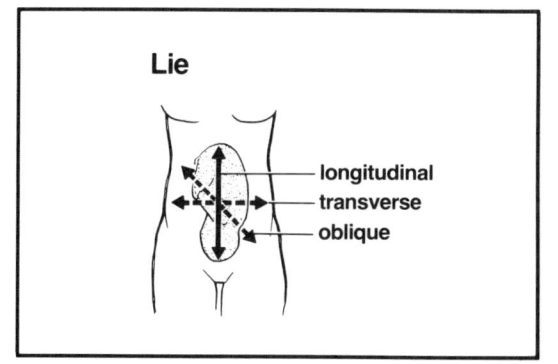

FLEXION

How your baby is flexed in your uterus will also affect his birth. In normal flexion, your baby's spinal column is bent forward, his chin is against his chest, and his arms are folded. His thighs are pulled up to the abdomen and the calves of the lower legs are against his thighs. In this flexion, your baby is about half as long as if he were completely stretched out.

POSITION

Position is determined by the placement of your baby's head in relation to your pelvis. For the purpose of describing the location of your baby in relationship to your body, your pelvis is divided into eight segments. There are three segments on your right-hand side and three segments on your left-hand side. The segment directly in back is called the direct posterior segment. The segment directly in front is called the direct anterior segment.

Three terms designate your baby's position. The first term, L or R (*l*eft or *r*ight), describes which segment of your pelvis your baby is turned to. The middle term, O, M, and S (*o*cciput, *m*entum, or *s*acrum), identifies your baby's presenting part—head (occiput), chin (mentum), or buttocks (sacrum). The last term, A or P (*a*nterior or *p*osterior), tells

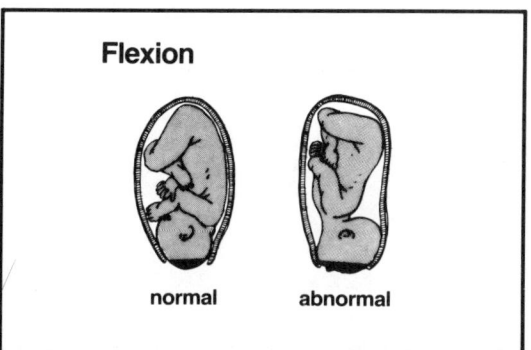

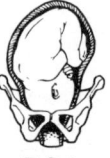
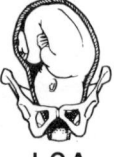

Anterior Positions

R.O.A.   L.O.A.

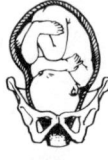
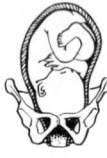

Posterior Positions

L.O.P.   R.O.P.

whether the presenting part of your baby is turned toward your backbone or pubic bone.

Anterior. The anterior position is the most common and most preferable since it requires the least amount of rotation before your baby is born. With the anterior position, you will probably be able to lie on your back comfortably with the head of the bed elevated. Your contractions will be felt primarily in your abdomen.

Posterior. The posterior position requires the greatest rotation and results in the longest labors and the most backaches. Contractions will probably be felt in your back, and they will have an irregular pattern of strength and length. As your baby is born, his head usually rotates into a position where the hard part of his skull will be pressing your tailbone and you may experience pain in your back.

PRESENTATION

Presentation describes that part of the baby which lies closest to the cervix. An optimum labor and delivery occurs when your baby lies with his head pointing downward in a vertex or cephalic presentation, thus forming an effective wedge for opening your cervix; his chin is tucked onto his chest so that the smallest diameter of the back of his head passes through first. When the back of his head is turned toward your pubic bone, the soft part of his face is against your tailbone, which is designed to yield to pressure.

Sometimes, because of the size or irregularity of your pelvis or the position of the baby, his head does not fit into your pelvis. When the buttocks of your baby comes first, the presention is called breech, and may cause problems during labor and birth.

Breech. There are several types of breech presentations. In a complete breech, the buttocks and legs are born first. Your baby's knees and hips are flexed. In a frank breech, the buttocks come first but the legs are straight with the feet up by the baby's head. A single or double footling breech occurs when one or both feet come first. When your baby is born in a kneeling position, it is called a kneeling breech.

Other presentations. A brow presentation is difficult for both the baby and the mother. A vaginal delivery of a shoulder presentation is impossible.

BABY'S MOVEMENTS DURING BIRTH

During labor the normal descent of your baby through the pelvis is a continuous process comprised of a series of turns and twists. Just as you might twist and turn your foot to get it into a boot, your baby passes through your inlet, through the diagonal conjugate of the passageway, and finally through the pelvic outlet.

Descent. To describe your baby's descent, an imaginary line is drawn across the ischial spines of your pelvis. This line is called station zero. The station number represents the descent of your baby from the pelvic inlet through the outlet. The inlet is designated as the minus five station. The ischial spines are at station zero. Once through the ischial spines, the baby passes through the plus stations in the birth canal.

Engagement. During your pregnancy, your baby's head may be floating above or dipping into your pelvic outlet. As the time for birth nears, he begins his descent into your pelvis. When the widest diameter of your baby's head has reached the level of your ischial spines at station zero, it is said to be engaged. Engagement often occurs in the last weeks of pregnancy with first babies, but in women who have had other babies, it may not occur until labor itself.

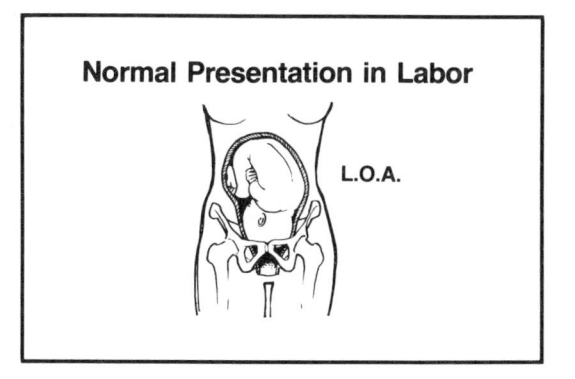

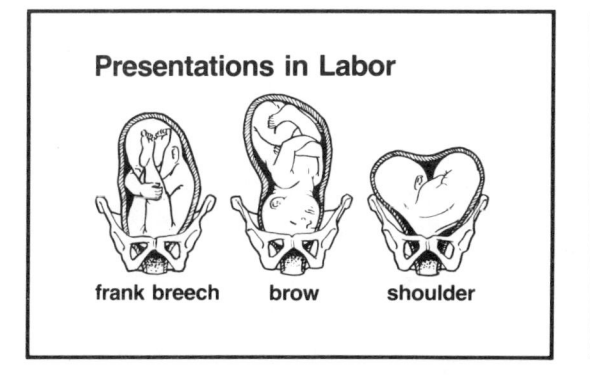

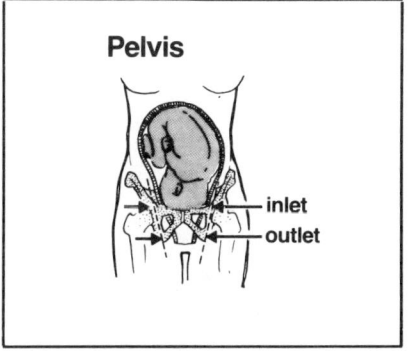

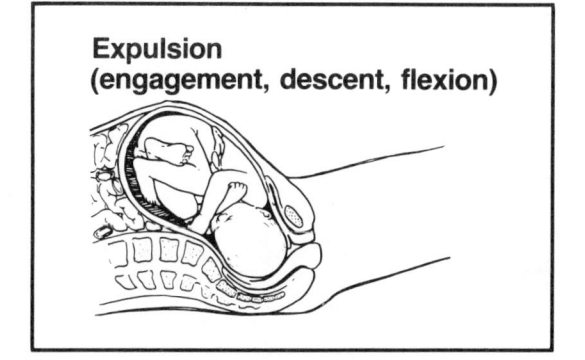

Normal Presentation in Labor

L.O.A.

Presentations in Labor

frank breech   brow   shoulder

Pelvis

inlet
outlet

Expulsion (engagement, descent, flexion)

Expulsion (internal rotation)

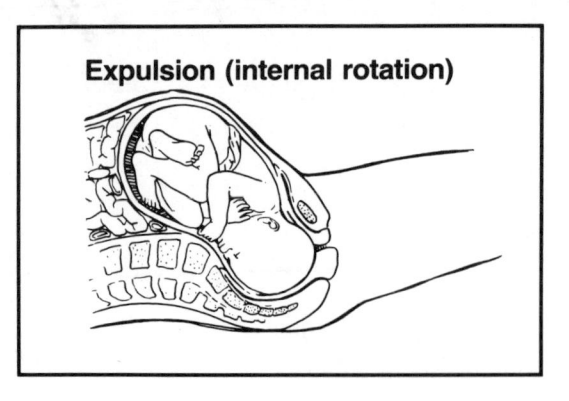

Internal rotation. An amazing phenomena of birth is your baby's rotation as he accommodates his head to the different diameters of your pelvic inlet and outlet. As your baby descends into the inlet, he turns his head to the side, facing your hip, so that his head will fit the greatest diameter of your inlet with ease. As he moves down the passageway into the outlet, he turns his face toward your back, making the greatest diameter of his head fit the greater front-to-back diameter of your pelvic outlet.

Extension. With his chin on his chest and his head flexed, the smallest part of your baby's head passes through your pelvic outlet. The back of his neck then lodges beneath your pubic arch, which acts as a pivotal point for the rest of his head. As the force of the contractions and your pushing efforts continue, your baby's head gradually lifts off his chest, with his neck extended. Your baby is usually born with his head facing down toward your back.

External rotation. After the emergence of his head, your baby remains facing down only a short time, and very soon turns his head to one side or the other of his own accord. This external rotation is due to the fact that his shoulders are turning sideways in your pelvis.

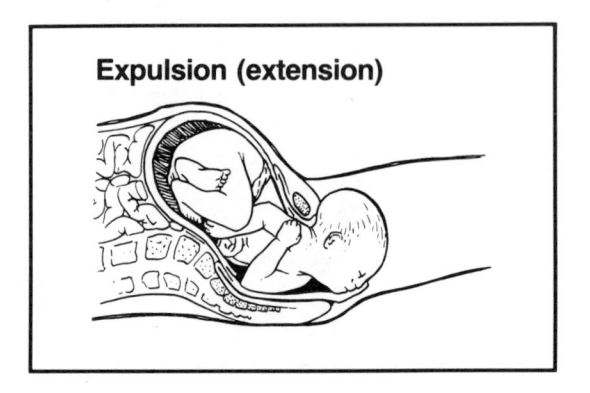

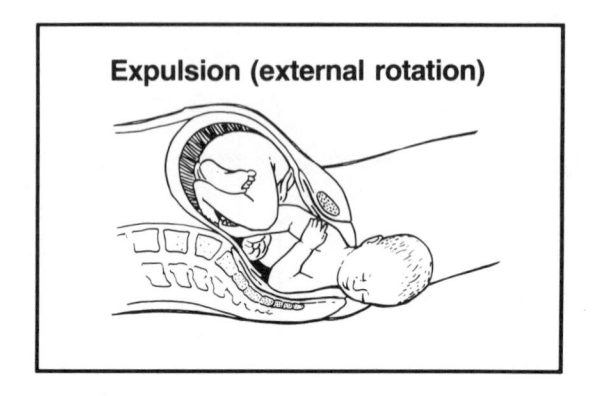

Expulsion (extension)

Expulsion (external rotation)

POWERS (CONTRACTIONS)

In most first pregnancies, the woman wonders how a baby can pass through such an obviously small opening. The whole function of the uterine contractions of labor is to open the cervix, from 0 to 10 centimeters, the diameter of your baby's head. Only after the cervix has opened does your baby pass through the expandable walls of the birth canal.

How Does a Contraction Feel?

Uterine contractions usually begin at the top of your uterus at the fallopian tubes and spread with decreasing intensity over the body of the uterus down toward the cervix.

As a contraction is starting, you will feel a slight hardening, or tightening, in your back or above the pubic bone, spreading toward the groin and covering your entire uterus. The uterus will become quite hard, remain tight for a few moments, then become progressively softer until it returns to its normal state. This may take from 30 to 60 seconds. The intensity of contractions change from a slight tightening at the beginning of labor to a much more rigorous feeling as labor progresses.

What Are Contractions?

Contractions are the means by which labor and delivery take place. During a contraction, the muscular fibers of the uterus tighten and shorten. The muscles in the uterus are involuntary; they contract and relax whether you want them to or not. When they contract, they shorten the fibers of the uterus and eventually thin out and take up the cervix into the uterine body. When they relax, the muscles do not return to their former length but become progressively shorter, thus reducing the uterine capacity after each contraction.

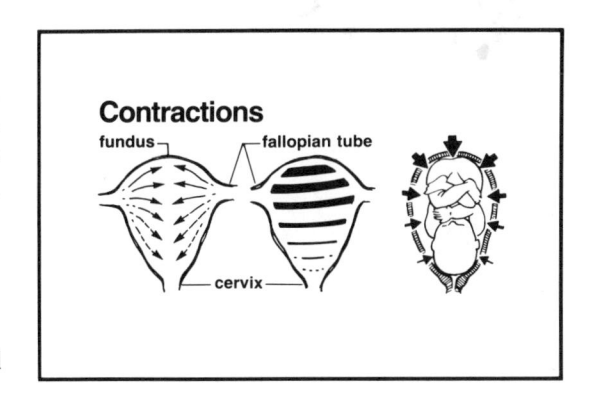

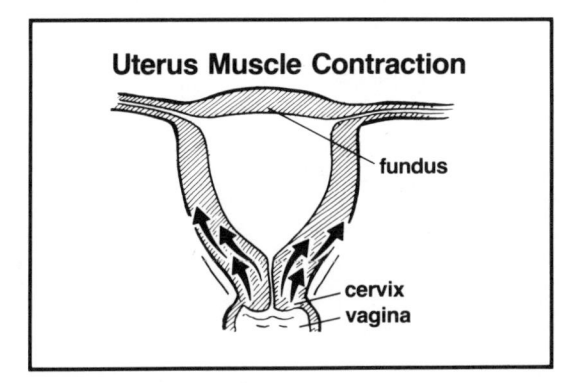

Uterus (effacement/dilatation)

- nonpregnant
- pregnant (at term)
- in labor (first stage)
- in labor (second stage)

Contractions

increment — peak — decrement — rest period

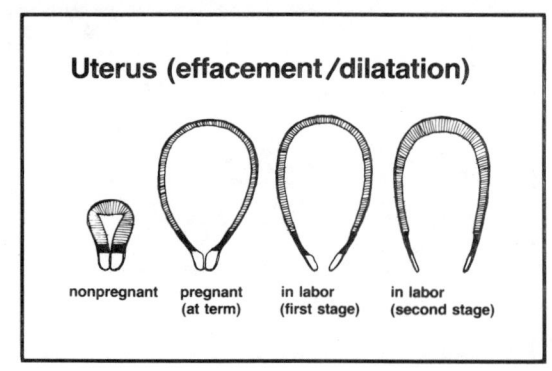

There are three important elements to each contraction: the duration, or how long it lasts from beginning to end; the frequency, or how long the interval is between one contraction and the next; and the intensity.

Contractions may last as few as 30 seconds during early labor to as long as 90 seconds in the latter phases of labor.

The interval between contractions gradually diminishes from about twenty minutes between each contraction during very early labor to ten minutes, five minutes, and finally two or three minutes during very active labor.

The intensity of early contractions may be so slight that you do not even know you are in labor. As labor progresses the strength of the contractions increases, and in the latter part of labor they can become extremely intense. During delivery the contractions are usually perceived to decrease in intensity.

Increment/Decrement

Each contraction has three parts: the increment (or buildup), the peak, and the decrement (or tapering off), with a rest period between contractions. The increasing and decreasing of a contraction is similar to the mounting and subsiding of a wave. It starts slowly, increases in intensity, reaches a crest, and then subsides. During labor it may be helpful to picture a contraction as an ocean wave—you can see it gathering, cresting, and subsiding.

Rest Periods or Intervals

Labor is a sequence of these contractions alternating with rest periods, or intervals between contractions. Even though labor may last 12 hours, you are really working only three to four hours of the time. These periods of relaxation not only provide rest for you and your uterine muscles, but are essential for your baby, preventing the contractions from interfering with his supply of oxygen.

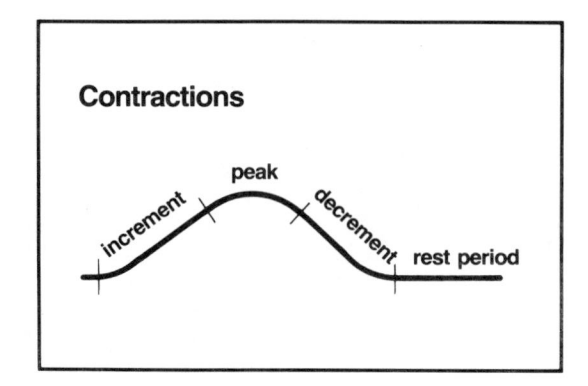

3.

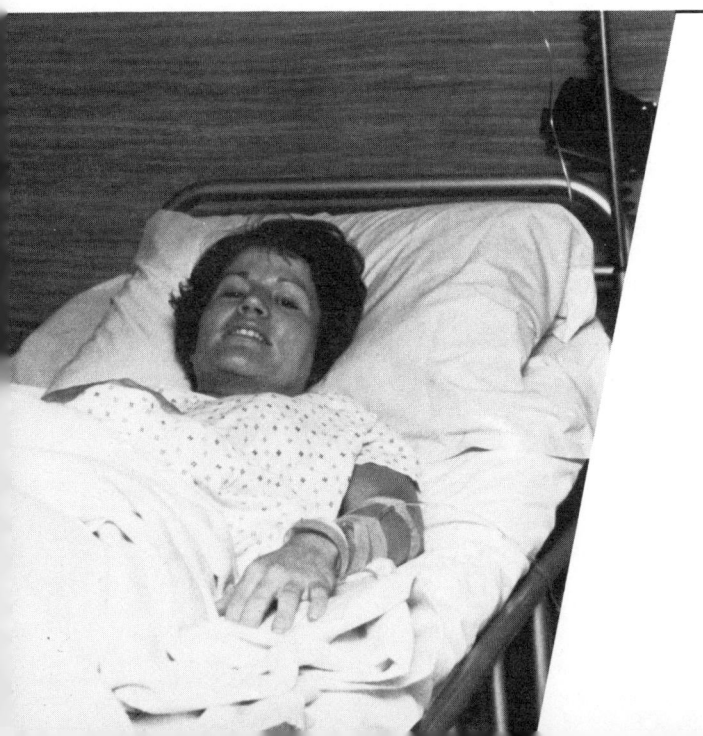

The Birth Process

Labor Curve (first labor)

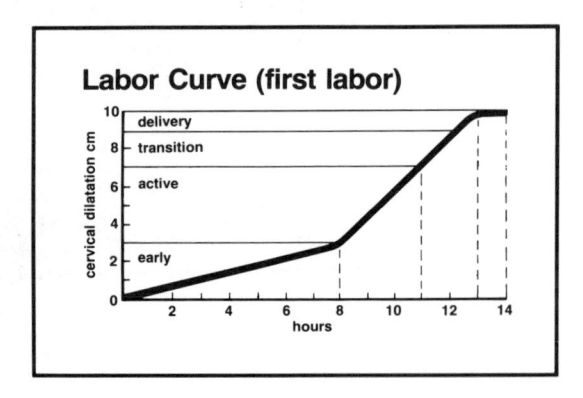

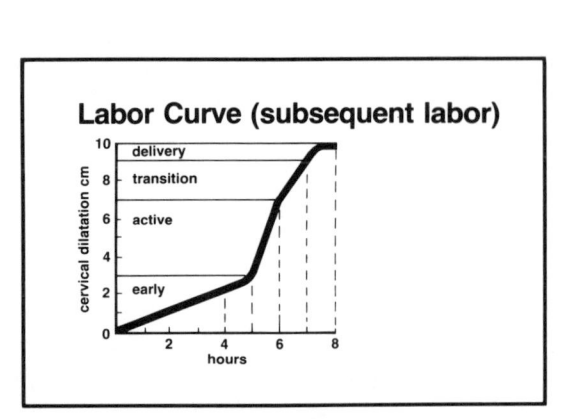

Your birthing attendants will talk about childbirth in terms of stages and phases. Each carries with it both physiological and emotional changes. It is important for you, the laboring mother, and you, the coach, to be aware of these changes as you cope with the increasing challenges you will experience during the birth of your child.

The whole process is divided into four stages. The first stage, labor, consists of opening the cervix. The second stage is the delivery of your baby. The third stage is the expulsion of the placenta, and the fourth stage, immediate postpartum, is the period immediately following birth.

Of all the stages of birth, it is the first stage, labor, that is the most demanding from the mother's and coach's point of view.

LABOR (FIRST STAGE)

In the first stage of birth the purpose of the contractions is to thin out (efface) and open (dilate) the cervix from 1 to 10 cm. If your labor lasts 12 hours, the first stage usually will take up the first 10 hours.

Effacement and dilatation are not processes separate from one another, but take place more or less together. Dr. E. A. Friedman studied the emotional and physiological patterns of women in labor. He found that for the majority of women, labor follows a regular pattern: early labor, active labor, and transition.

Dr. Friedman developed a graph that showed these phases of labor for women experiencing their first labor. Another graph shows that women who are experiencing second or subsequent labor may expect a shorter labor and delivery.

Labor Curve (subsequent labor)

Early Labor

For a woman having her first baby it usually takes many hours for her to progress through effacement to 3-cm. dilatation. This phase is called early, or latent, for the progress is slow and almost imperceptible.

During early labor, a time of excitement and emotional adjustment for the mother, the contractions cause the effacement and dilatation of the cervix to about 3 or 4 cm. Contractions during effacement cause the tissues of your cervix to be pulled into the body of the uterus so that the internal and external cervical openings become one and the uterus opens right into the vagina. Once this is accomplished, the contractions combined with the force of your baby's head pushing against the cervix begin to dilate it.

The early contractions and effacement may take place weeks before true or active labor begins. The contractions are relatively weak and last from 30 to 60 seconds, with irregular intervals in between. With your first baby, partial effacement usually takes place before dilatation; with later babies it may take place at the same time as dilatation.

Active Phase

From about 3 to 7 cm., the contractions dilate the cervix much more quickly. Progress is fast and very obvious. The contractions become more intense in their efforts to open the cervix from 3 to 7 cm. With each succeeding contraction, the cervix opens a bit more to create an opening large enough to permit the passage of your baby's head. This is called the active phase of labor.

The contractions increase in duration and intensity as the cervix dilates. They usually last about 60 seconds, with a rest interval of 1–3 minutes between contractions. Early and

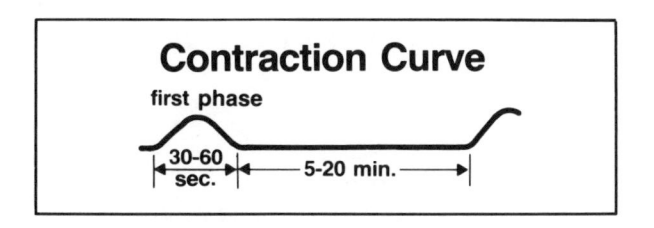

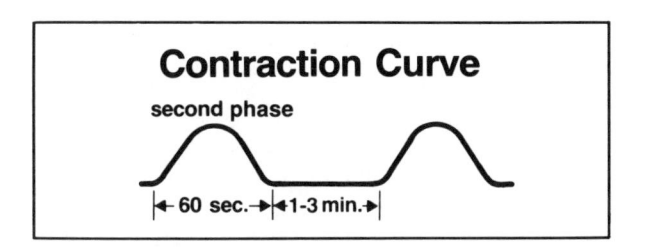

Contraction Curve
first phase

|← 30-60 sec. →|← 5-20 min. →|

Contraction Curve
second phase

|← 60 sec. →|← 1-3 min. →|

active phases usually last from 5 to 9 hours with the first baby. For women who have had other babies, it usually takes from 2 to 5 hours.

Transitional Phase

At about 7 to 8 cm., there is a plateau. This phase is commonly known as the transitional stage, because of the change in the nature and quality of contractions and in the emotional changes the laboring mother undergoes.

Although the cervix is not fully dilated during this phase, the expulsive efforts of the uterus begin to exert their influence, and at this stage the woman may have an overwhelming desire to push. In addition to becoming longer and stronger, the contractions become extremely intense. They can last anywhere from one to two minutes with little rest in between. Transition is the hardest part of labor and it helps to remember that it usually lasts for only a short time, as little as five to ten minutes and sometimes as long as an hour.

DELIVERY (SECOND STAGE)

Once the cervix is completely open and the baby has entered the birth canal, the contractions seem to decrease in intensity and a new force comes into play. The uterine con-

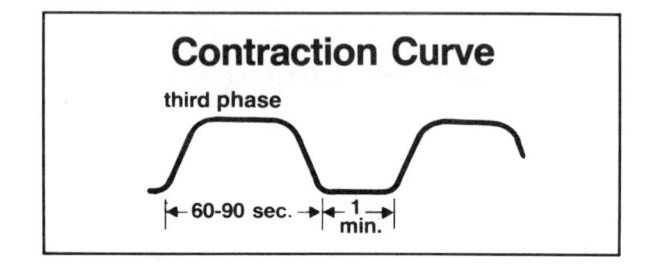

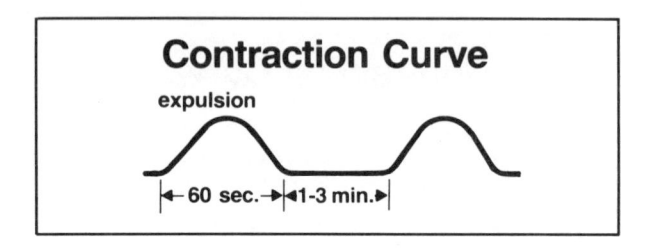

Contraction Curve
third phase
60-90 sec. | 1 min.

Contraction Curve
expulsion
60 sec. | 1-3 min.

tractions are combined with the mother's pushing with her abdominal muscles to expel the baby from the uterus. The baby descends down the birth canal, under the pubic bone, through the pelvic floor, and out the external opening.

The contractions during this stage last about 60 seconds, with rest periods of 1–3 minutes between contractions. The entire expulsion stage usually takes from about 30 minutes to 2 hours.

PLACENTAL DELIVERY (THIRD STAGE)

The contractions do not stop with delivery. The moment your baby is born, the sudden shrinking of the uterus helps detach the placenta from the uterine wall. Further contractions help clamp down the uterine blood vessels. Within the next several minutes, contractions will cause the placenta to become completely detached and delivered through the vagina.

It is important that the placenta is delivered intact and that no part of it remains in the uterus to cause hemorrhaging or complications. The placenta will be carefully examined both where it was attached to your uterus and where it was attached by the umbilical cord to your baby.

IMMEDIATE POSTPARTUM (FOURTH STAGE)

Immediate postpartum begins with the birth of your baby and continues for the first hour afterward. During this time, the beautiful moments of bonding and becoming attached take place. The doctor and attendants are concerned with stabilizing the mother's vital signs and assuring her body's healthy return to the nonpregnant state. The birthing attendants carefully monitor the mother's blood pressure and blood flow to ensure against hemorrhaging.

Duration of Labor

	1st labor	other labors
effacement and dilatation	12 hrs.	7 hrs. 20 min.
expulsion	1 hr. 20 min.	3 min.
placenta	10 min.	10 min.

CONCLUSION

As far as your work is concerned, the progress of a normal fourteen-hour labor and delivery can be compared to climbing a mountain.

On a fourteen-hour hike, the first eight hours of early labor compare with easy hiking on grassy meadows. The slope is gradual and it is pleasant to stop and smell the flowers and feel the warm sun on your body.

In the next four hours of active labor, you begin the climb into the foothills and this requires more effort. You stop talking and start concentrating on the work you have ahead of you.

The next hour, transition, you find yourself on the face of the mountain, wondering why you ever came and how you got into this. Your partner is behind you supporting you, guiding you, and helping your every step. Your labor ends (delivery) with your arrival at the peak, and you are suddenly aware of the magnificence and beauty of your efforts at the unforgettable moment of the birth of your child.

The last hour after your arrival on the top of the mountain is spent in recovery and rest and enjoyment of your accomplishment.

4.

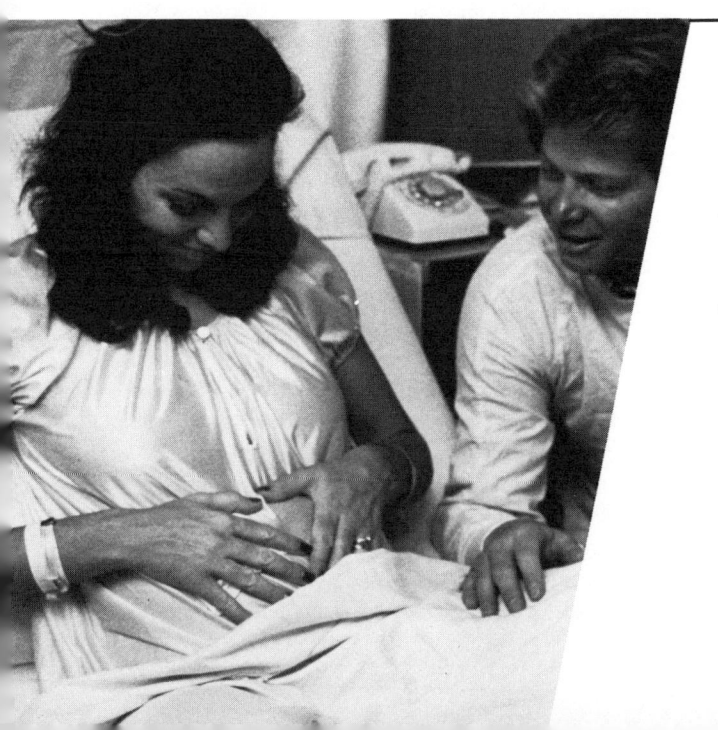

Alleviating Pain in Childbirth

Anyone who is pregnant or who plans on becoming pregnant is concerned with how she is going to react to labor and delivery. Stories brought to us from the Bible through modern literature combined with stories shared by family and friends perpetuate the concept of pain in childbirth.

We do know that there are some very real factors that may cause pain in childbirth. We also know that a woman who goes into labor with a high level of anxiety and with high expectations of pain will probably suffer a more painful experience, a longer labor, and more complications than a woman who goes into labor with a low level of anxiety, low expectation of pain, and tools and techniques to cope with her contractions.

As a prepared woman you will interpret your contraction as the mechanism to deliver your baby and as a signal to begin your work. You will respond to each contraction with controlled breathing and relaxation. During labor, your threshold of pain will be raised by concentrating on a focal point, breathing patterns, relaxation, and massage.

Prepared childbirth relies on the participation of a trained coach, who is most often the husband but who can be a close friend or birth attendant. Your role as a coach is to direct the mother's concentration toward her breathing and relaxation techniques, to give verbal encouragement and directions. These, combined with massage and stroking, will be of tremendous importance to the mother's comfort.

Since childbirth can be a traumatic experience you must practice the techniques at home to make them an automatic response to the contractions you will experience during labor and delivery.

There are three basic factors that may cause discomfort in childbirth. Physical factors such as the intensity of uterine contractions and the stretching and tearing of tissues during labor and delivery may cause pain. Emotions such as anxiety and fear may lower the threshold of pain and cause the laboring woman to perceive her uterine contractions as more painful than they might otherwise feel. Finally, normal physiological functioning of the uterus and muscles may be impaired by excessive muscular tension and improper breathing, resulting in pain in the muscular tissues of the body.

What kinds of tools and techniques do you need for alleviating or eliminating these factors in childbirth? Which of the physical causes of pain cannot be altered and must be

Neuromuscular Control

	untrained woman	trained woman
stimulus	contraction	contraction
interpretation	pain	signal to begin work
response	tenses, holds breath	controls breathing, relaxes

brain- interprets selects

body- responds

uterus- contracts

dealt with? What are the emotional factors that can be dealt with? And what physiological factor can be avoided?

PHYSICAL FACTORS

Uterine contractions are the mechanism that opens the cervix and expels the baby. Effective contractions are essential and desirable parts of a normal labor and delivery. You do not want to change the length, strength, and duration of the contractions, but you can understand and learn to cope with them by using distraction, breathing, relaxation, massage, and effleurage to diminish your perception of their intensity.

EMOTIONAL FACTORS

Anxiety, fear, and feelings of isolation and panic are all common emotions during childbirth. Unfortunately, these feelings can translate themselves into very real physical sensations of pain and fatigue. Anxiety and tension constrict your blood vessels and cut down on the vital oxygen supply you and your baby need. These normal feelings can be intensified by ignorance, isolation, and sense of being out of control. On the other hand, anxiety can be remarkably diminished by preparation before birth, which includes getting information on what is going to happen to your body and why, and how you are going to feel. Feelings of isolation are diminished by knowing that you have an educated coach and supportive staff. When you go into labor with tools and techniques to help you cope with contractions, feelings of being out of control are replaced by feelings of competence.

PHYSIOLOGICAL FACTORS

Tension during childbirth counteracts the effectiveness of contractions and prolongs labor. Excessive muscular tension and improper breathing not only inhibit the contractions but may cause oxygen starvation of the working uterus, resulting in toxicity and pain in the uterine muscle itself, along with the muscles of the rest of your body. Tension and improper breathing patterns (such as holding your breath or overbreathing) can cause exhaustion, a lowered threshold of pain, or hyperventilation. These factors can be prevented through relaxation and breathing techniques. Relaxation will help keep you refreshed and give you a feeling of well-being. Proper breathing will oxygenate all of your muscles, keep you from hyperventilating, and keep you in control.

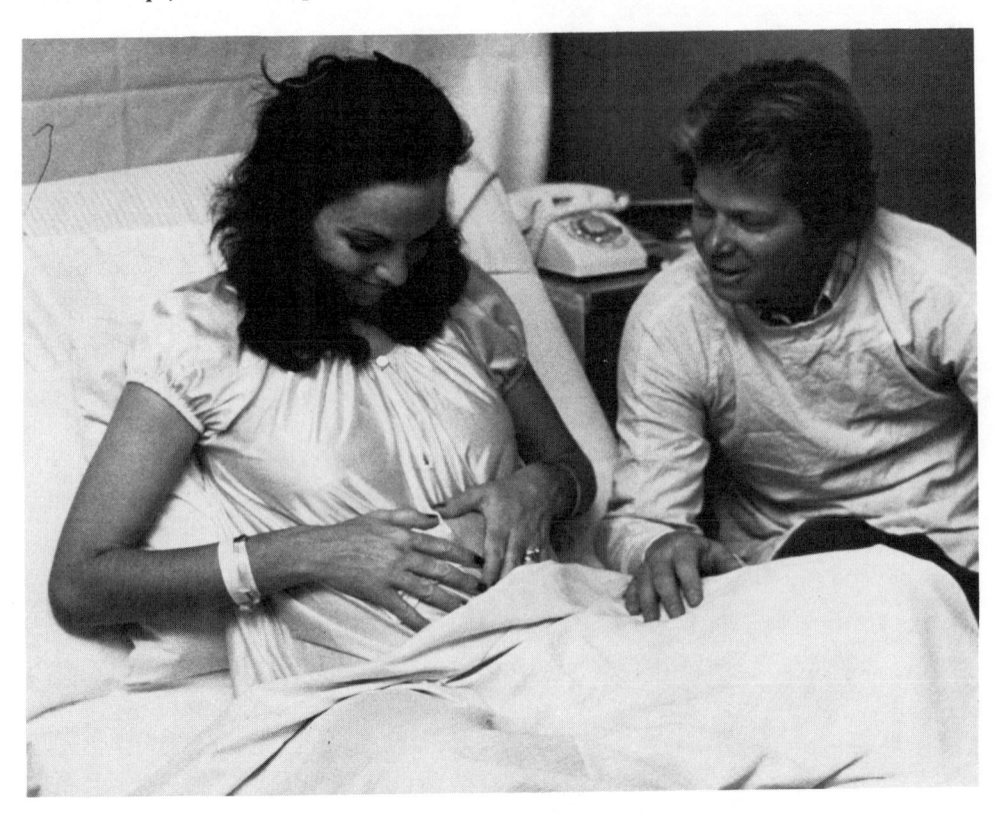

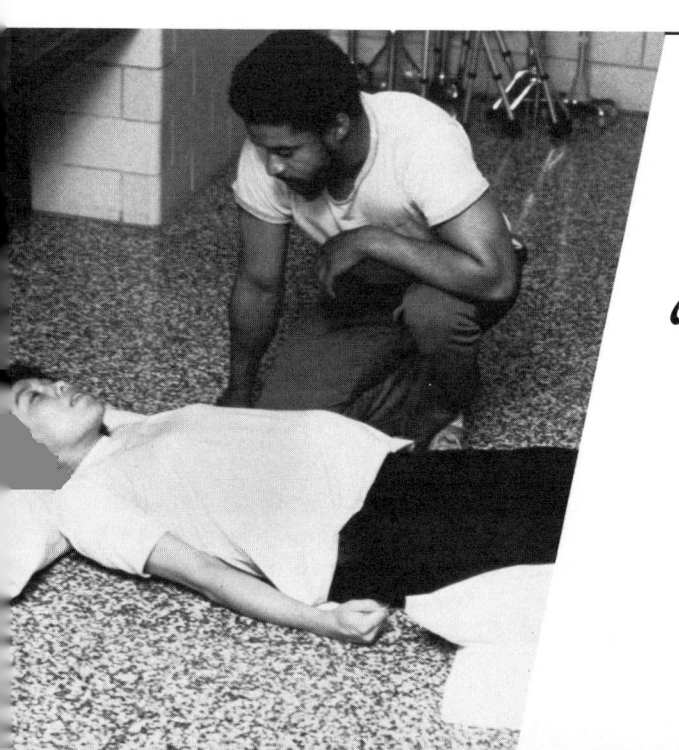

5.
Controlled Relaxation and Concentration

During labor and delivery, relaxation is one of your most important techniques. Research shows that relaxed, less anxious mothers haver shorter labors and deliver babies with higher APGAR scores (the APGAR scale measures newborns' respiration, color, heart rate, and responses). Relaxation not only shortens your labor, but conserves your energy, decreases pain, allows your contractions to be more effective, facilitates the oxygen supply to you and your baby, and prevents the fear/tension/pain cycle from taking over.

Two hormones affect contractions. The hormone oxytocin causes the uterus to contract. When you are tense, another hormone called adrenalin is produced, counteracting the effect of oxytocin and making your contractions less effective. Thus excessive tension can actually prolong labor.

Another important factor during labor is the large amount of oxygen your uterus needs. If your muscles are tense, constricting your blood vessels, the circulation of oxygen is impaired, causing muscle fatigue and pain. Contraction of blood vessels also results in decreased circulation and decreased oxygen supply to your baby.

Knowing how to relax during labor will help you remain calm. You will be able to communicate more effectively with the people who are supporting you. You, the laboring mother, and your coach will enjoy a greater sense of being in control. Your threshold of pain is raised and your perception of the intensity of the contraction is diminished if you practice controlled relaxation at the onset of a contraction. When a woman actively relaxes with her contraction, rather than fighting it, she consumes less energy. She is much less fatigued and has more energy available to meet the physical demands of her labor.

RELAXATION EXERCISES

Although relaxation is a natural state for human beings, in the hustle and bustle of our society the majority of people seem to have lost the art long before adulthood. Once you relearn relaxation, you have an important gift that you can use for the rest of your life, and that you can hand down to your children as well.

The following exercises will take you through a relearning process:

1. total relaxation—how it feels for your body to be tense, and how it feels to be relaxed
2. progressive relaxation—how to control parts of your body both in tension and relaxation
3. touch relaxation and the technique of stroking—relaxing with the help of your coach's touch
4. neuromuscular control—how to relax parts of your body while other parts are under tension

Setting Up

All relaxation exercises should take place in a room that is well ventilated and at a comfortable temperature. Turn off the radio and lights and shut out any other bothersome external stimuli. Take the phone off the hook. Take off your shoes, wear loose clothing, and empty your bladder before you begin.

POSITION

Find a position, lying on your bed or on the floor or sitting in a comfortable chair, where you can relax comfortably and completely for the next fifteen minutes. To avoid lying flat on your back, you may wish to assume a side-lying position. Do not cross your feet or legs. Flex your arms and legs so that you are sure to get good circulation to all parts of your body. Check to see that there are no pressure points on your body. To help you feel more comfortable, use pillows to support all parts of your body: under your head, around your abdomen, under your arms and legs.

BREATHING

A slow, deep, comfortable breathing pattern will help you relax. Learn to take in a slow, deep breath through your nose. As you inhale, concentrate on breathing in warm, moist, relaxing air, feeling it spread throughout your body. As you exhale through your mouth, concentrate on breathing out all remaining tension in your body. With each breath you take, concentrate: inhale warm, relaxing air; exhale all tension out.

CONCENTRATION

Concentration, a major part of relaxation, will help raise your threshold of pain. The first part of your relaxation exercises, in which you learn how to relax your whole body and become aware of its parts, concentrates on experiencing freedom from tension. The second part of your neuromuscular exercises, in which you learn how to relax parts of your body while other parts are under tension, concentrates on total muscle control.

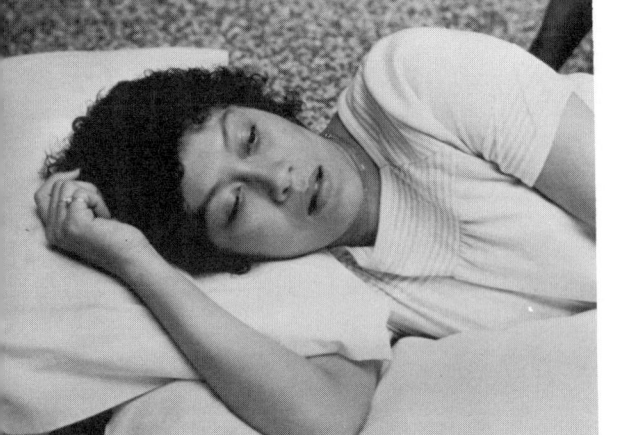

Total Relaxation

The first stage in relaxation teaches you to become aware of each and every muscle in your body and release tension to attain total body relaxation.

Step 1: Position. For the first step in complete relaxation it is important to check again that you are in a position where you can relax comfortably and completely. Now, close your eyes and take the next five minutes to learn to know your body. Make yourself as calm and peaceful as possible.

Step 2: Five deep breaths. Take in a deep breath and let it out. Take in a second deep breath of warm, relaxing air and, as you let it out, feel the tension flow out of your body. Take in another deep breath and feel the warm, relaxing air seep into your body; as you let it out, concentrate on releasing tension in your body. Take in a fourth deep breath and let your body relax even more. As you let it out, concentrate on the tension flowing out of your body. Take in a fifth deep breath and let your body flow even more into relaxation. As you exhale, let all of the tension flow out of your body, making it even more relaxed.

BODY AWARENESS

Now that you are so completely relaxed, take a few moments to mentally check each part of your body. Feel how good it is to be relaxed. Concentrate on feelings of relaxation.

- Starting at your scalp, concentrate on relaxing every muscle of your face: cheeks, eyes, tongue, mouth, and jaw.
- Relax your throat and neck muscles.
- Relax all tension in your shoulders; let them flow into the surface beneath you.
- Relax your arms, making them feel as heavy as possible.
- Let your hands and fingers go as limp as possible.
- Relax your chest and abdominal muscles.
- Relax your spine; feel the relaxation flowing from vertebra to vertebra. Relax the muscles in the small of your back.
- Let your buttocks go flabby, let them flow into the surface beneath you.
- Relax your pelvic floor muscles.
- Release all tension in your thighs; let them go limp.
- Relax your calves and feel them flow into the surface beneath you.
- Release all tension in your ankles and feet and feel it flow out of your toes.
- When you feel completely relaxed, take in five more breaths and with each breath make your body more relaxed.

VISUALIZATION AND IMAGERY

Visualization and imagery may help you relax. Relax the muscles of your body by thinking of such phrases as:

Limp as a rag doll
Floating like a cloud
Floating like a leaf on the ocean
Light as a feather

Heavy and sinking
Flowing like sand onto a beach
Limp as a piece of spaghetti
Warm and melting like butter

Every time you practice, try to get your body more relaxed than it has ever been. It is important to enjoy your daily session.

Progressive Relaxation

The goal of progressive relaxation is to learn how it feels to have your body completely tensed and then, in contrast, completely relaxed.

Step 1: With your body completely relaxed, concentrate on feeling each relaxed muscle in your body. Make each part even more relaxed: scalp, eyes, cheeks, tongue, jaw, throat, shoulders, chest, upper arms, elbows, lower arms, fingers, spine (vertebra by vertebra), abdomen, buttocks, thighs, knees, calves, feet, and toes.

Step 2: Now, tense your whole body from top to bottom: squint your eyes, clench your teeth, tense your whole face and throat, bring your shoulders up, tense arms, clench your hands and fingers, tense your chest, pull in your abdomen, squeeze your buttocks, bring your thighs together, tense your calves and point your toes up toward your knees (don't point your toes downward or you may get a cramp). Hold and concentrate on each muscle and how it feels to be tensed. After holding tension, oxygen deprivation can cause real pain in your muscle tissue.

Step 3: Carefully release the tension in each muscle from the top of your head to your toes. Concentrate on how good it feels for a muscle to be out of tension and in a relaxed state.

Step 4: Do this five times. Concentrate on being aware of every part of your body. Concentrate on learning to identify the feelings that accompany tension and relaxation.

BODY AWARENESS

Now, instead of feeling your total body tensed and then relaxed, you are going to learn to isolate muscles and feel different parts under tension and different parts under relaxation. You will concentrate on tensing and releasing each individual part of your body until you can tense and release each muscle at will. As you practice you will become more and more adept at controlling your body.

Step 1: Tense your face: scalp, eyes, mouth, and cheeks. Hold and feel tension. Release. Concentrate on how these muscles feel in a relaxed state.

Step 2: Tense your throat and shoulders (pull them up toward your ears). Hold and feel tension. Release. Concentrate on how these muscles feel in a relaxed state.

Step 3: Tense your chest and back (pull your shoulders together in front of you). Hold and feel tension. Release. Concentrate on relaxing spine, vertebra by vertebra. Notice how these muscles feel in a relaxed state.

Step 4: Tense your abdomen (pull in your tummy). Hold and feel tension. Release. Concentrate on how these muscles feel in a relaxed state.

Step 5: Tense your buttocks and pelvic floor (squeeze buttocks together and pull up on pelvic floor). Hold and feel tension. Release. Concentrate on how these muscles feel in a relaxed state.

Step 6: Tense your thighs and calves. Hold and feel tension. Release. Concentrate on how these muscles feel in a relaxed state.

Step 7: Tense your feet and toes (point your toes up toward your knees). Hold and feel tension. Release. Concentrate on how these muscles feel in a relaxed state.

Step 8: Tense your whole body once more. Hold and feel tension. Release your whole body. Concentrate on how your body feels in a relaxed state.

Touch Relaxation and Stroking

Touch relaxation will add another dimension to your ability to release tension. It is an important technique that you and your coach will use during your labor and delivery.

It consists of the coach's touching, with warm, firm, comforting hands, and the woman responding by releasing her tension toward the touch.

POSITION

The coach and the mother should be in a comfortable position. The mother may be semi-sitting with pillows under her head, shoulders, and knees, side-lying, or sitting in a chair. She should loosen her clothing and take off her shoes.

STROKING

The mother's role is to concentrate on allowing all the tension to flow into the coach's hands. As you feel his hands pass over your body, concentrate on releasing or letting go to the coach's touch. Feel tension flow out of your body with the stroking movements.

The coach's hands will bring important relief and comfort to the mother in labor. Think of your hands as one of the most important comforting tools that you have. Think of them as warm, gentle, firm, pleasing, solacing, easing, reassuring, and tender. Warm your hands by rubbing them briskly together before you place them on the skin of the woman. Place both hands gently on each side of the mother's thigh or shoulder. Then, with firm, gentle, long, and continuous downward movements, stroke over the thigh, knees, calf, foot, and out the toes (stroke from the shoulder over the upper arm, elbow, lower arm, hands, and out the fingers). Concentrate on feeling all of the woman's tension flow into your hands.

PRACTICE

1. *Mother:* tense whole leg and foot. *Coach:* with firm rhythmical touch, stroke down the thigh into the knee, calf, foot, and out through the toes. *Mother:* Release each part and concentrate on letting all tension flow into the coach's hands.

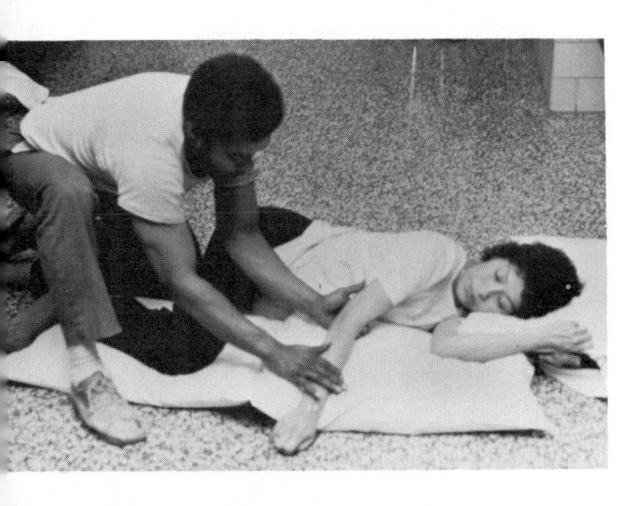

2. *Mother:* tense shoulder, arm, hand, and fingers. *Coach:* stroke down over the shoulder, down the upper arm, over the elbow, down the lower arm, and out through the hand and fingers. *Mother:* release each part and concentrate on letting all tension flow into the coach's hands.

3. *Mother:* tense neck, face, eyes, mouth and cheeks. *Coach:* stroke down over the forehead, eyes, cheek, mouth and neck. *Mother:* release each part and concentrate on letting all tension flow into the coach's hands.

4. *Mother:* tense spine and buttocks. *Coach:* stroke down over the spine and buttocks. *Mother:* release each part and concentrate on letting all tension flow into the coach's hands.

The coach should ask the woman if the stroking was helpful. Would she like it firmer? softer? gentler? harder? higher? lower? Her needs will change throughout her labor and the coach must monitor what is working most effectively and be able to change his techniques as her needs change.

Selective Relaxation (Neuromuscular Control)

It is unusual to have part of your body in tension and part in relaxation. However, when you are in labor, the involuntary muscles of your uterus will contract completely on their own. You cannot make them contract nor can you stop them from contracting. One of the difficulties you will meet in labor is that with part of your body in tension, the rest of your muscles will naturally want to tense also. Unfortunately, this tension will not only counteract the effectiveness of your contractions and prolong your labor, but it will also cause you pain and discomfort.

With selective relaxation you learn how to counteract this tendency by relaxing parts of your body while others remain tense. You practice contracting one set of muscles to simulate the contracting uterus, while at the same time you concentrate on making other parts of your body relax. These exercises are called neuromuscular exercises because they involve the interrelationship between your brain and your muscles.

You, the mother, concentrate on relaxing, or on releasing tension, in the part your coach has indicated. With your eyes open, concentrate on the parts of your body that are relaxed, making them sink deeper and deeper (or heavier and heavier; deeper and heavier; or any other imagery word that works best for you). Your aim is to concentrate on the muscles in which you are trying to release all tension, not the tensed muscles. Practice your deep, relaxed breathing (inhale warm, relaxing air; exhale out all the tension) with your relaxation. When your coach adds the stroking, be sure you concentrate on letting all remaining tension flow into his hands.

The coach gives directions for the mother to tense and relax parts of her body. You give her verbal commands: for example, tense your right arm and relax your left arm and both legs. When you are sure that she has relaxed each part to her maximum ability, you then stroke the relaxed parts of her body to help her relax even more.

SIMULATION

During practice sessions the coach can simulate the tension of a contraction by applying firm, even pressure with his fingers on the muscle area above the mother's knee or elbow. Gradually increase the pressure (mounting of the contraction), hold it (apex of the contraction), and then gradually decrease the pressure (as the contractions lets off). The mother must concentrate on relaxing all the other parts of her body.

CHECKING RELAXATION

The coach should check relaxation by gently picking up the mother's relaxed arm or leg in one of your hands, and gently turning it back and forth with the other hand. Checking at the place where it is attached to her body (either at the shoulder or hip), you will see it gently rock back and forth. You will feel it limp and heavy. Never touch the tense part to check tension, because in labor the mother should associate your touch only with relaxation.

Head, neck, shoulders: Gently move her head from side to side. You should feel no resistance.

Arms: Lift the arm with one hand, holding it with your other hand at the wrist and elbow. You should feel no resistance. The arm should feel heavy and the hand and fingers relaxed. It should be loose at the shoulder joint.

Legs: Lift the leg at the knee and ankle. The leg should feel heavy and the foot relaxed. It should be loose at the hip joint when you move it from side to side.

If any part feels tense, the coach should tell the mother to let all the weight just flop into his hands. Tell her to let it go completely heavy—and then heavier—into your hands. Or, you can tell her to let it go limp—and then more limp—into your hands. Find the word that is most effective for her. If she can't get it right away, be patient. Tell her it takes time and you will both work at it over the weeks. Tell her the harder she has to work at it during practice the more prepared she will be for the tremendous effort and concentration she will need during labor and delivery. Don't let her get tense over relaxing! Keep giving her encouragement and support.

EXERCISE I: ONE PART TENSED, ONE PART RELAXED

1. *Coach:* "Contract your right arm:" *Mother:* Tense your arm, shoulder, elbow, and fist, and raise your arm, holding it straight before you a couple of inches off the floor. *Coach:* "Relax your left arm and both legs." *Mother:* Concentrate on relaxation, not on tension. *Coach:* Check the relaxed parts, then add stroking to the left arm and both legs.
2. *Coach:* "Contract your left arm." *Mother:* Tense your arm, shoulder, elbow, and fist, raising your arm before you. *Coach:* "Relax your right arm and both legs." *Mother:* Concentrate on relaxation. *Coach:* Remind mother to concentrate on relaxed parts. Only stroke right arm and both legs; never touch the tensed arm.
3. *Coach:* "Contract your left leg." *Mother:* Tense your thigh, knee, foot, and toes. Be careful to point your toes toward your knee to avoid cramps. Keeping your thigh flat on the surface, bend leg at knee and raise foot and toes a few inches. *Coach:* "Relax your right leg and both arms." *Mother:* Concentrate on relaxation. *Coach:* Check relaxation. Stroke right leg, both arms.

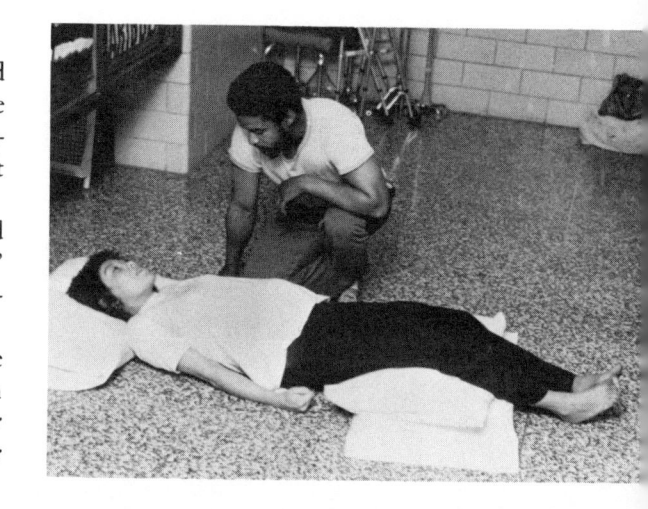

4. *Coach:* "Contract your right leg." *Mother:* Tense your thigh, knee, foot and toes. Leaving thigh on the surface, bend leg at knee and raise calf and foot a few inches off the surface. *Coach:* "Relax your left leg and both arms." *Mother:* Concentrate on relaxation. *Coach:* Check relaxation. Stroke left leg, both arms.

EXERCISE II: TWO PARTS TENSED, TWO PARTS RELAXED

1. *Coach:* "Contract your right leg and right arm." *Mother:* Tense and lift right leg and right arm. *Coach:* "Relax your left leg and left arm." *Mother:* Concentrate on relaxation. *Coach:* Check relaxation. Stroke left leg and left arm.
2. *Coach:* "Contract your left leg and left arm." *Mother:* Tense and lift left leg and left arm. *Coach:* "Relax your right leg and right arm." *Mother:* Concentrate on relaxation. *Coach:* Check relaxation. Stroke right leg and right arm.
3. *Coach:* "Contract both arms." *Mother:* Tense and lift both arms. *Coach:* "Relax both legs." *Mother:* Concentrate on relaxing both legs. *Coach:* Check relaxation. Stroke both legs.
4. *Coach:* "Contract both legs." *Mother:* Tense and lift both legs (bend at knee, raise foot). *Coach:* "Relax both arms." *Mother:* Concentrate on relaxing both arms. *Coach:* Check relaxation. Stroke both legs.

EXERCISE III: OPPOSITES TENSED, OPPOSITES RELAXED

This last part of the neuromuscular exercises is intended to increase the woman's power of concentration and relaxation even further. Since the right side of the brain controls the left side of the body, and vice versa, this exercise requires even more effort and concentration, which prepares her for the great concentration and control she will need to relax her body against the intensity of the contractions she will experience during labor.

1. *Coach:* "Contract your right arm and left leg." *Mother:* Tense your arm and leg. *Coach:* "Relax your left arm and right leg." *Mother:* Concentrate on relaxation.

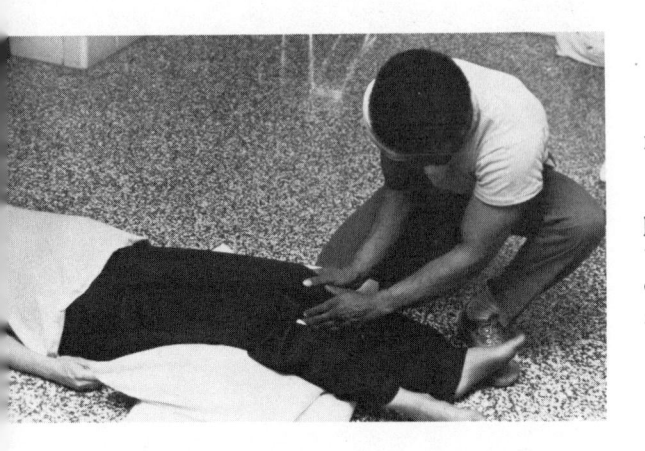

Coach: Check relaxation. Stroke left arm and right leg.
2. *Coach:* "Contract your left arm and right leg." *Mother:* Tense your arm and leg.
   Coach: "Relax your right arm and left leg." *Mother:* Concentrate on relaxation.
   Coach: Check relaxation. Stroke right arm and left leg.

Don't be disappointed if you have more difficulty with this exercise than you have had with others. This takes more effort, more control, and more concentration. The harder you work at attaining control and concentration, the more you will be prepared to handle the actual contractions of labor.

Daily Practice Schedule

Your conscious relaxation techniques will be an important response to the intensity of contractions during childbirth. Because controlled relaxation is probably going to be one of your most difficult tasks, it is important that you practice it twice daily beginning in your seventh month of pregnancy. Practice with your coach so that you become accustomed to automatically responding to his directions and touch.

Practice the following schedule twice daily: once in morning alone, once in evening with coach, using touch relaxation and stroking techniques:

1. Total relaxation: body awareness, visualization
2. Progressive relaxation: (tense and relax parts)
3. Neuromuscular exercise control (exercises I, II, III)

CONCENTRATION

Concentration on a focal point helps raise your threshold of pain and decreases your perception of the contractions' intensity. The beginning of a contraction will be your signal to concentrate on a focal point and begin your breathing and relaxation techniques.

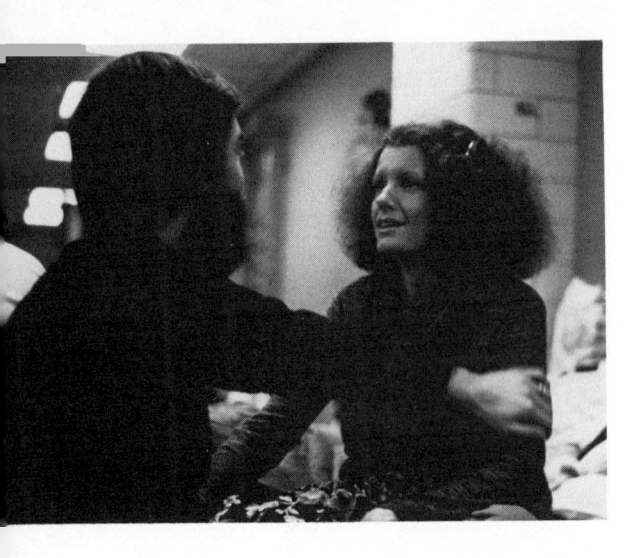

Procedure

For the focal point you may choose either an object already in the room (such as a clock or picture) or a colorful and pleasant object of your own that has some personal meaning and which you can bring with you (such as a picture, an art object, a photo of someone you love); or, you may choose your coach's face on which to focus.

Whatever you choose, be sure it is placed at a comfortable distance so that you will not strain your eyes looking at it over a long period of time. During labor you will use this object as a point of concentration as each contraction begins. Your eyes should be open and focused in a comfortable and relaxed position. As the contraction begins, focus on the point and use it to center all of your concentration as you begin your breathing and relaxation. Avoid staring until your focus blurs; concentrate on keeping your facial muscles relaxed.

As your labor progresses, your ability to focus may change and you may want to bring the focal point closer to you. You will also want to move the object as you change position. Remember to adjust the focal point to allow your eyes to be in a relaxed position.

6.

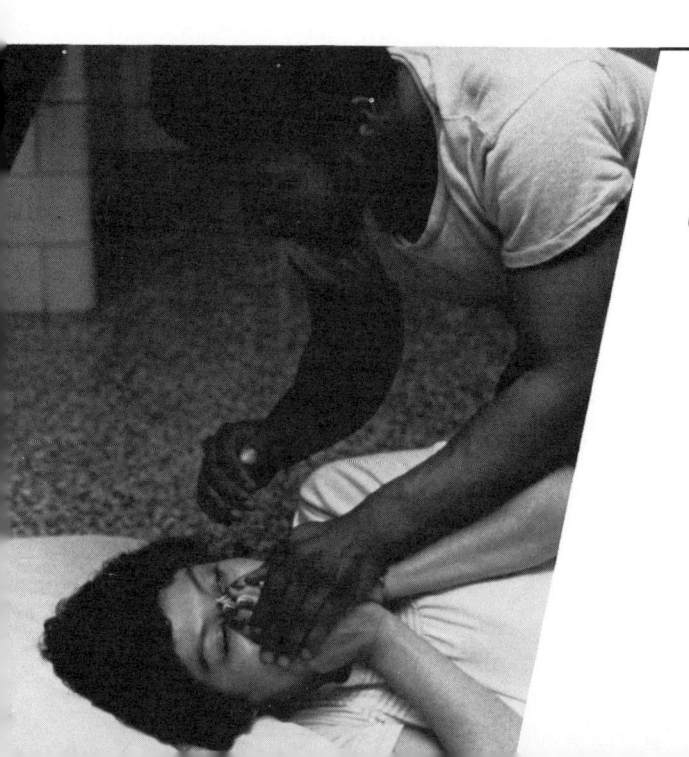

Controlled Breathing

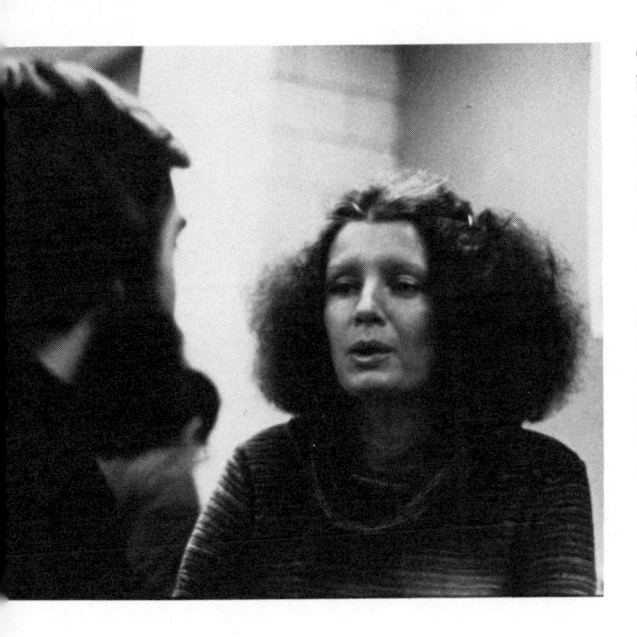

Controlled breathing is an essential element of prepared childbirth. Although deep breathing is a natural response to a contraction, when labor becomes pronounced, many women tense up, hold their breath, clench their teeth, or scream. These actions are in direct conflict with your contractions and can cause exhaustion, prolonged labor, pain, and discomfort. Controlled breathing aids in relaxation and provides important oxygen to your baby.

The uterine contractions of labor and delivery are powerful and use a lot of oxygen. Your muscles need oxygen to be effective. Controlled breathing patterns provide the oxygen your uterine and other muscles need for a normal, efficient labor. Breathing can be an active response to your uterine contractions. Concentration on your breathing will help diminish your perception of the contractions' intensity and will keep a balanced amount of oxygen and carbon dioxide in your system. Controlled breathing patterns help the laboring woman not only to work with each contraction but to take advantage of rest periods in between, leaving her more rested and refreshed.

When you breathe in (inhale), oxygen goes into your lungs. When you breathe out (exhale), carbon dioxide is released. Between your lungs and the contents of your abdomen is a thin, flat, disc-shaped muscle called the diaphragm. As you inhale, your lungs fill your chest cavity, pushing your diaphragm down. When you exhale, your lungs are emptied and the diaphragm comes up.

When you inhale, breathe in through your nose; when you exhale, breathe out through your mouth. Breathing in through your nose allows warm, moist, filtered air to come into your lungs, and also helps keep your mouth from becoming dehydrated. Because many pregnant women experience swelling of mucous membranes, they find it easier to exhale through their mouths.

As the intensity of labor increases it is not uncommon for a woman to begin a type of fast, uneven breathing that leads to hyperventilation and tension, and eventually to lack of control. The breathing patterns you will learn are designed to help you keep your breathing natural, even, rhythmic, quiet, and comfortable so that you will remain relaxed and in control of your labor.

To ensure maximum efficiency, remember the following points:

1. Use the focal point, relaxation, and concentration techniques with your breathing patterns.
2. Begin and end each pattern with a cleansing breath, which will signal to your coach the beginning and ending of each contraction.
3. Reserve the use of each breathing level for the time when it is absolutely necessary.
4. Make each inhale and exhale as even as possible so that there is an adequate balance of oxygen and carbon dioxide.
5. Whatever breathing pattern you are using to match the intensity of your contractions, be sure it is comfortable. It should not be labored or exhausting but at an even, quiet rate that suits you.
6. Every woman has her own natural rate of breathing (be it slow, fast, or somewhere in between). The rate of breathing in each pattern should fit your needs, and the coach should take care not to superimpose his own rate of breathing (which might be quite different), but to adjust his speed and rate to the needs of the laboring woman.
7. Finally, the woman in labor should remember that with each inhalation she should concentrate on taking in warm, relaxing air—and with each exhalation she should consciously practice releasing tension.

Remember, there is no one right way to breathe, just as there is no one right way to labor. Every woman must find and adjust to her own pattern that keeps her comfortable and relaxed. Any other pattern will end in feelings of breathlessness, suffocation, and finally, hyperventilation.

Coach's Role

Help the woman remain relaxed and refreshed. Remind her not to start the controlled breathing until she absolutely has to. Help her stay with the slow chest breathing as long as possible, but proceed to the next stage of breathing when she needs it. Match the intensity of the breathing to the intensity of the contractions. Remind her to consciously relax with each exhalation and to concentrate on her breathing.

BREATHING PATTERNS

Cleansing or Signaling Breath

Each contraction begins and ends with a cleansing or signaling breath. This breath becomes a conditioned response to the beginning and end of contractions and informs your coach of the progress of the contraction. The inhalation signals you to begin your concentration and the exhalation is a conditioned cue for you to relax. The cleansing breath begins by a slow inhalation of air through your nose with your mouth closed, expanding your lungs to a comfortable degree. The air is exhaled through slightly pursed lips, allowing a comfortable return to normal.

First-Level Breathing (Deep, Slow)

First-level breathing is designed to meet the intensity of your contractions during the early part of labor. These early contractions are mild, with rest periods in between. Your breathing response to these contractions is a comfortable, relaxed, and deep slow chest breathing.

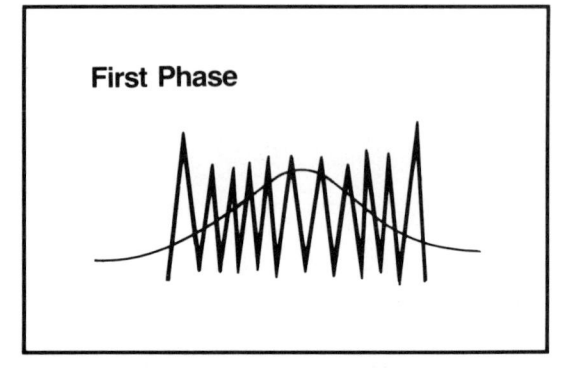

First Phase

TECHNIQUE

Begin in a relaxed position. Concentrate on your focal point. Practice a contraction that lasts sixty seconds. Take in a deep cleansing breath and let it out. Inhale by breathing in a smooth, even stream of air through your nose, and then exhale by breathing out a smooth, even stream of air through slightly pursed lips. Usually, six to nine breaths per minute are comfortable, though you must explore your own rate. Your aim is a slow and steady natural pace, not speed. Be sure that the breath you take in and the breath you let out are even, to maintain the balance of oxygen and carbon dioxide in your system. It may be helpful to pace your deep chest breathing by counting "one, two, three, four, five" as you inhale and "one, two, three, four, five" as you exhale. Continue this pattern until you get the rhythm and speed that are natural and comfortable to you.

PATTERN

Contraction begins: Take in a deep cleansing breath and exhale
Contraction mounts: Inhale (count in five); exhale (count out five); continue through end of contraction
Contraction ends: Take in a deep cleansing breath and exhale

Second-Level Breathing (Shallow Accelerated/Deep Slow Combination)

As your labor progresses the intensity of your contractions increases. They are longer, their apex is stronger, and you will have less of a rest period in between. Slow chest breathing is not adequate to match the intensity of the apex and you will now need to add another type of breathing that is shallow and more active.

TECHNIQUE

Shallow breathing keeps your diaphragm up off your uterus. A gradual buildup in the speed of breathing matches the intensity of the contractions. This breathing pattern is characterized by a light, shallow breathing in and out of your mouth at the peak of the contraction. This rhythm of breathing helps you remain relaxed, provides adequate oxygen, and adds to your concentration.

Practice the light, shallow breathing as follows: Tilt your head back slightly to allow free passage of air through your throat. Put your tongue behind your upper teeth to keep your mouth from getting dry. Now silently say the sound "hee." Feel where the air comes in on your upper palate. This is where you will do your light breathing. Match the peak of your contraction with a series of short shallow breaths. Visualize counting "in one" and "out one" so that you establish a rhythmic and controlled pattern. It may help you to imagine the sound "hee" as you practice the shallow breathing. The rate is usually around twenty to thirty breaths a minute. If you get out of breath, or feel as though you are suffocating, slow down.

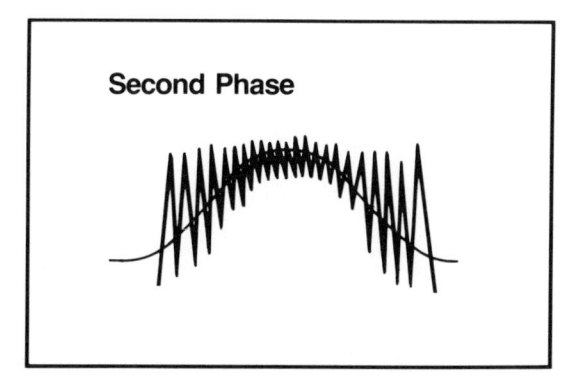

Combined breathing (deep slow and shallow accelerated). Now that you have the tools of deep and shallow breathing, it is time to coordinate them and work with the intensity of the contraction. Practice with a contraction that lasts sixty seconds. As your contraction starts, take in a signaling breath and exhale. Start with your deep slow breathing. As your contraction mounts, match it with increasingly shallower breathing. This should sound like a train leaving the station. When the contraction reaches its apex, open your mouth, and with your tongue behind your upper teeth, begin a light, silent, rhythmic "hee" breathing. As the intensity of the contraction lets up, return to your deep breathing, which sounds like a train pulling into a station. When the contraction eases off, take a deep cleansing breath to signal its end.

PATTERN

Contraction begins: Take in a cleansing breath and exhale

Contraction mounts: Breathe in through nose and out through mouth; breathe in 4 counts, breathe out 4 counts; breathe in 3 counts, breathe out 3 counts; breathe in 2 counts, breathe out 2 counts

Contraction apex: Tilt head back with tongue behind teeth, open mouth, and switch to shallow accelerated breathing (silently say "hee, hee, hee" throughout the apex); continue accelerated breathing (or panting) throughout apex

Contraction lets off: Breathe in through nose 2 counts, breathe out through mouth 2 counts; breathe in 3 counts, breathe out 3 counts; breathe in 4 counts, breathe out 4 counts; breathe in 5 counts, breathe out 5 counts

Contraction ends: Take in a cleansing breath and exhale.

Use counting until you are accustomed to the pattern and rate. You may or may not find counting helpful in labor.

Variations

Always remember to match the intensity of your breathing with the intensity of the contractions. Your contractions during labor may not resemble the textbook contractions you have read about. Some begin slowly, reach an apex, let off, and, without warning, piggyback with another contraction. You have the tools to work with the intensity of your contractions. Practice matching your breathing patterns to these variations.

Contraction Variations (60 seconds)

normal   early
late   prolonged
piggyback

EARLY PEAK CONTRACTIONS

Contraction begins: Take a deep signaling breath and exhale
Contraction mounts quickly to apex: Switch to light accelerated breathing
Contraction continues at apex: Continue light accelerated breathing
Contraction begins to decline: Change to deep slow breathing
Contraction lets off: Continue deep slow breathing
Contraction ends: Take a deep cleansing breath and exhale

LATE PEAK CONTRACTIONS

Contraction begins: Take in a deep cleansing breath and exhale
Contraction mounts slowly: Begin deep slow chest breathing
Contraction increases: Slightly accelerated deep breathing
Contraction reaches apex: Switch to shallow accelerated breathing
Contraction apex continues: Continue shallow accelerated breathing
Contraction ends: Take a deep cleansing breath and exhale

PROLONGED PEAK CONTRACTIONS

Contraction begins: Take in a deep cleansing breath and exhale
Contraction reaches apex quickly: Switch to shallow accelerated breathing

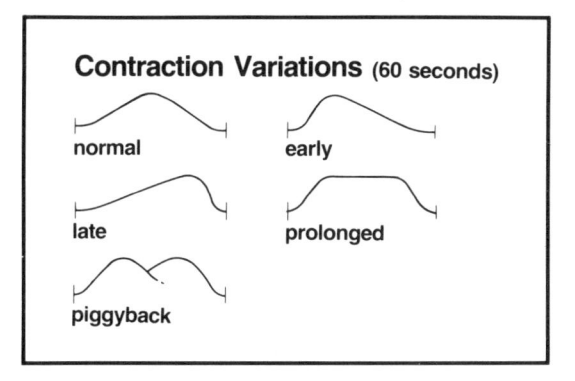

Contraction apex continues: Continue shallow accelerated breathing
Contraction ends: Take a deep cleansing breath and exhale

PIGGYBACK CONTRACTIONS

Contraction begins: Take a deep cleansing breath and exhale
Contraction mounts: Begin deep slow chest breathing
Contraction reaches apex: Switch to shallow accelerated breathing
Contraction begins to decelerate: Switch back to slightly accelerated deep chest breathing
Contraction begins to mount again: Switch to shallow accelerated breathing
Contraction lets off: Change to deep slow breathing
Contraction ends: Take a deep cleansing breath and exhale

Third-Level Breathing (Transition)

Deep slow and shallow accelerated breathing will take you through your labor up to the transition phase. The contractions during transition are extremely strong with long peaks and may be difficult to manage. They can last anywhere from sixty to ninety seconds, with only short intervals between. Pushing at this time, before the cervix is completely dilated, may result in injury to the cervix. One more breathing technique will help you resist the urge to push: The transitional pant/blow.

TECHNIQUE

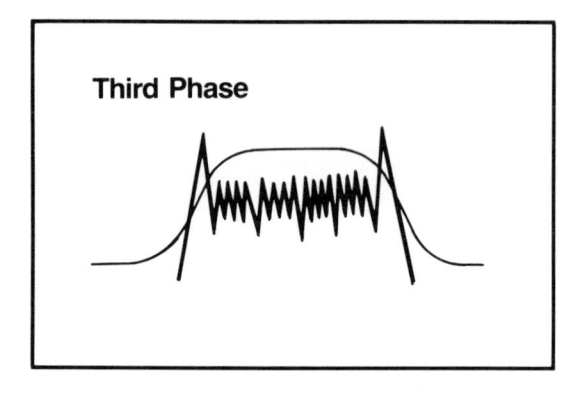

The breathing during transition utilizes the shallow accelerated breathing that you have learned, with one important addition: a short blow interspersed throughout the contraction at the end of three shallow breaths. The short blow helps counteract the desire to push. It may be described as a short puff of air (sounding like "hoo!" or "whew!") escaping from your cheeks, much as you would blow out a candle or blow on a feather. It may help you to imagine the sounds "hee, hee, hee, hoo" as you practice. Again, this breathing is as slow, even, comfortable, relaxed, and rhythmical as possible to meet your individualized needs. Practice transitional breathing for a contraction that lasts ninety seconds.

PATTERN

Contraction begins: Take in a cleansing breath and exhale
Contraction mounts: Switch to light, accelerated breathing: inhale, exhale; inhale, exhale; inhale, exhale; inhale and give a short puff or blow (or, "hee, hee, hee, hoo! hee, hee, hee, hoo! hee, hee, hee, hoo!"); continue to end of contraction
Contraction ends: Take in a cleansing breath and exhale

VARIATIONS

If your contractions during transition are long and extremely intense at the apex, you may find relief in using two short pants and a blow ("hee, hee, hoo!") or even a pant/blow pattern ("hee, hoo!").

Contraction begins: Take in a cleansing breath and exhale
Contraction mounts: Inhale, exhale; inhale, exhale; inhale, blow ("hee, hee, hoo! hee, hee, hoo! hee, hee, hoo!"); continue to end of contraction. OR: Inhale, blow; inhale, blow; inhale, blow ("hee, hoo! hee, hoo! hee, hoo!"); continue to end of contraction
Contraction ends: Take a cleansing breath and exhale

When the transition period is almost over, the intensity of the contraction and the desire to push at the apex are overwhelming. At this time it may give relief to blow, blow, blow at the apex and return to the two- or three-pant pattern after the apex, beginning and ending with a cleansing breath. NOTE: You do not have to use the "hee" and "hoo" sounds; use them only if they help you.

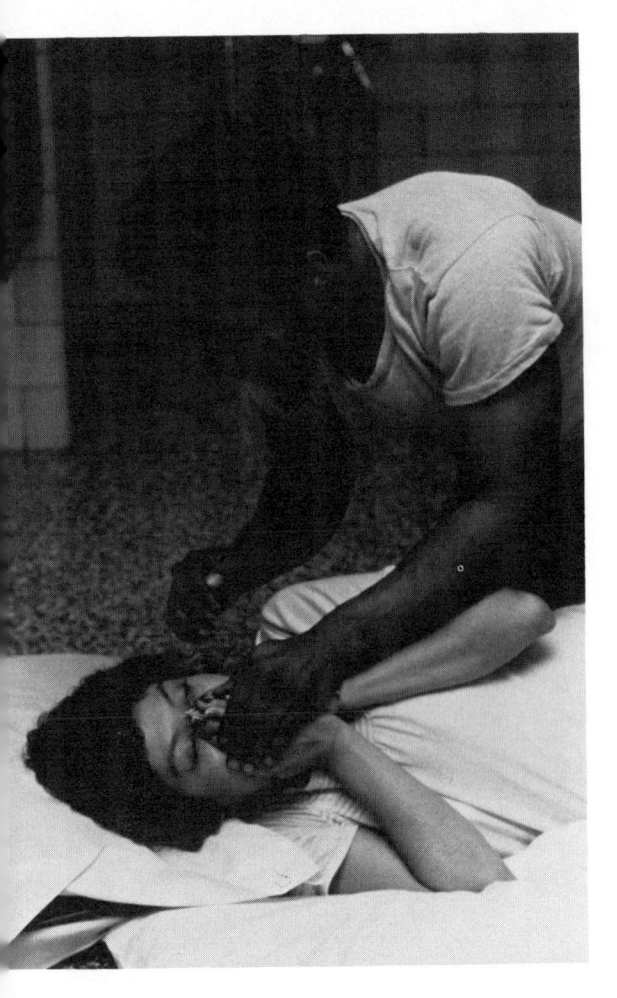

Hyperventilation

Hyperventilation can result from an imbalance of oxygen and carbon dioxide in your system. Uneven breathing patterns, breathing too rapidly, and tension are all possible causes. Watch for the symptoms of hyperventilation: lightheadedness, dizziness, tingling and numbness in your face or hands. Should you experience any of these, first cup your hands over your nose and mouth and breathe into them to let your system balance itself. Hold your breath for a few seconds after the contraction is over. If this does not work, hold a paper bag over your mouth and nose and breathe into it until the symptoms disappear.

Finding Your Style

There is no one breathing technique that is going to work perfectly for every woman in labor and delivery. Breathing techniques are only effective if, and when, they work for you. Everyone must find the pattern and style that fits her individualized needs.

There are several ways to find the style that is right for you. Keep your breathing pattern *simple;* don't get so caught up with complex patterns that you forget to use breathing techniques in labor and transition. Your breathing style must be *comfortable,* for if you feel you are going to suffocate, or that you are not getting enough air, it won't work for you in labor. There is no right number of breaths per minute for everyone; you must practice until you find the individual rate that works for you. You may even find that you will have to change that rate in labor. If you breathe too fast, you will feel that you are suffocating. If you breathe too loudly, you will become exhausted. If you breathe unevenly, you will become hyperventilated. If you start your breathing too early in labor, it will lose its effectiveness.

Remember to keep your breathing rate at a slow, comfortable speed. Concentrate on keeping an even, rhythmical pattern. Keep your controlled breathing as quiet as possible, and don't start your controlled breathing techniques in labor until you absolutely have to.

Coach's Checklist

To help direct the mother in finding the most effective rhythm for her, ask her the following after a contraction:

- Slow—Ask her if her breathing is at a comfortable natural pace.
- Even—Ask her if her breathing is even, to ensure balance.
- Rhythmic—Ask her if she has found her rhythm; if not, help her count (at her rate, not yours).
- Individualized—Ask her if she feels short of breath or hyperventilated. If so, help her slow her breathing down and count with her to make it even.
- Comfortable—Ask her if she feels comfortable, or is tense and short of breath. Help her to relax her throat and shoulders. Slow her breathing down.
- Relaxed—Ask her if she feels relaxed. Remind her to concentrate on breathing in warm, relaxing air and breathing out tension with each exhale. Stroke her body.

Daily Practice Schedule

Your controlled-breathing technique will be your conditioned response to your contractions during childbirth. That means you must practice it daily before you go into labor so that it will be an automatic response during labor and delivery.

Practice the following schedule twice daily, once in morning alone and once in evening with coach.

1. Practice first-level contraction breathing
2. Practice second-level contraction breathing: average contraction and variations (late, early, prolonged, and piggyback)
3. Practice transitional breathing
4. Practice expulsion breathing

Combine with your relaxation, focal point, and effleurage techniques (see pages 66–67).

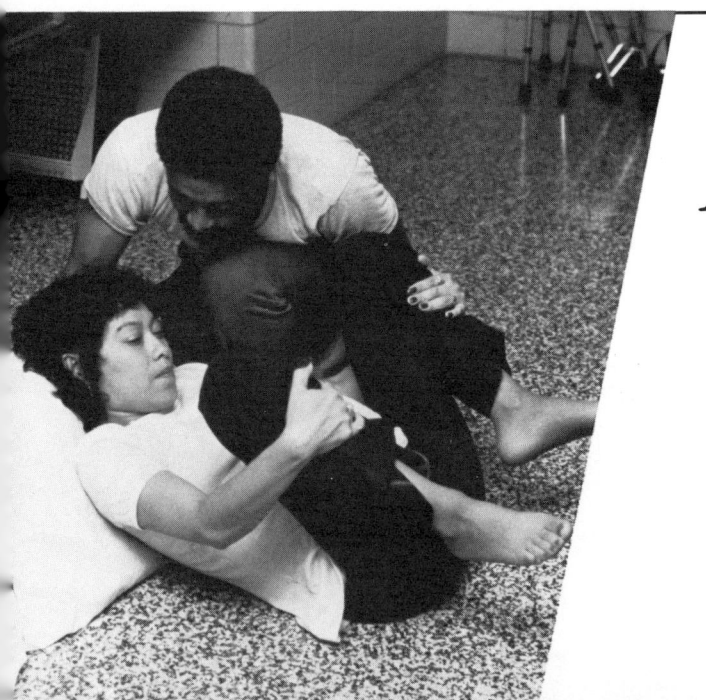

7.
Expulsion Techniques

POSITION

Women have long delivered their babies in a squatting position. Only in relatively recent times have mothers delivered their babies while lying on their backs. The best childbirth position in regard to effective pushing is squatting. The chin is off the chest, shoulders are rounded, arms bent and out, back curved and pelvis tilted. These body dynamics can be translated and adapted into any pushing position you choose, whether sitting, semi-sitting, or side-lying.

Concentrate on keeping your head erect and your shoulders rounded. The small of your back should be straight and your pelvis tilted. Bring your legs up to both sides of your uterus. Relax your perineum and pelvic floor.

SEMI-SITTING

To assume a semi-sitting labor position, place pillows under your knees to give them comfortable flexed position and enough pillows behind your head and back to partially lift you up. The small of your back should be pressing against the bed.

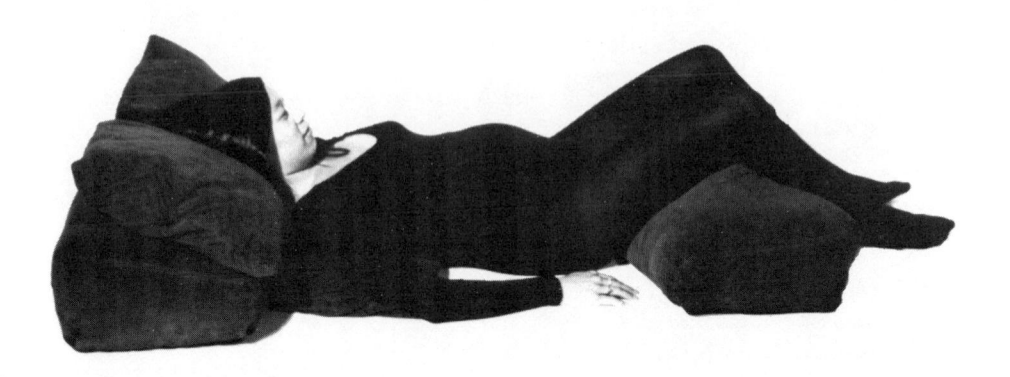

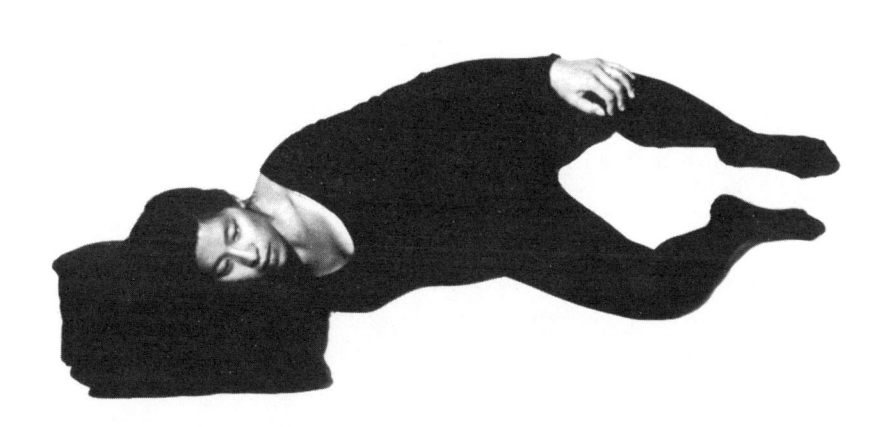

SIDE-LYING

Lying on your side during expulsion takes the weight of the uterus off your back. Extend your lower leg and place over bent upper leg on a pillow. Support your whole body with pillows. The side position is effective for expulsion because contractions are more efficient and give the least amount of sensation.

PRACTICE

Assume the squatting position to get the feel of your body, and then, if you prefer, change to the side-lying or semi-sitting position. Choose the position that is most comfortable for you and surround yourself with pillows to support your back, legs, and arms. (Your coach will support your shoulders and head at a natural angle that will not cut off your air or make you uncomfortable.)

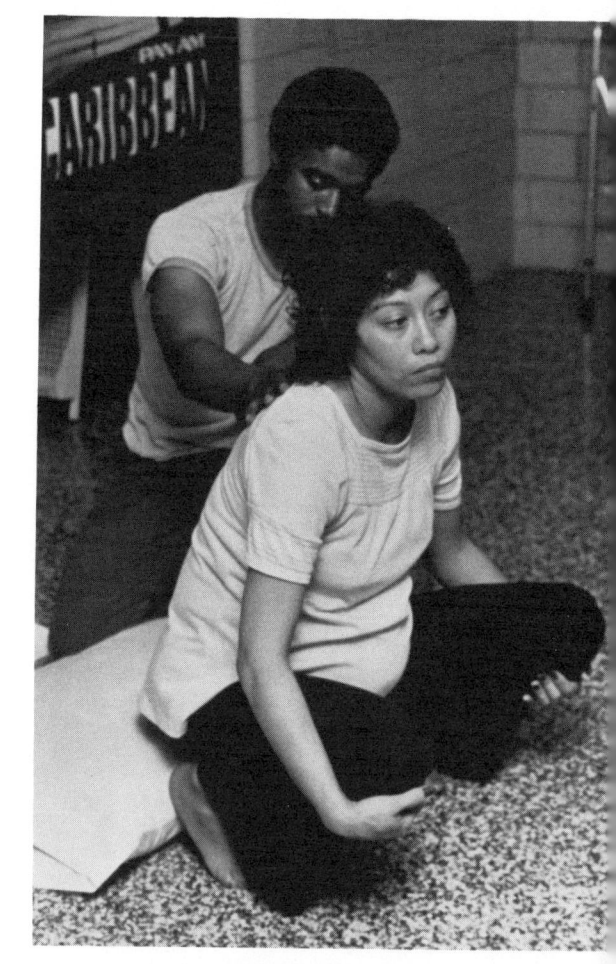

PUSHING

Pushing effectively with your abdominal muscles does not mean pushing as having a bowel movement, which contracts the lower muscles and makes pushing less effective. You use the same upper abdominal muscles you used for the "blowing out the candle" exercise (see pages 54–55). To be most effective you must not only concentrate on pushing down and out with your abdominal muscles but on relaxing all other muscles, especially your pelvic floor, thighs, and perineum. Remember to relax your face, jaw, throat, and shoulders.

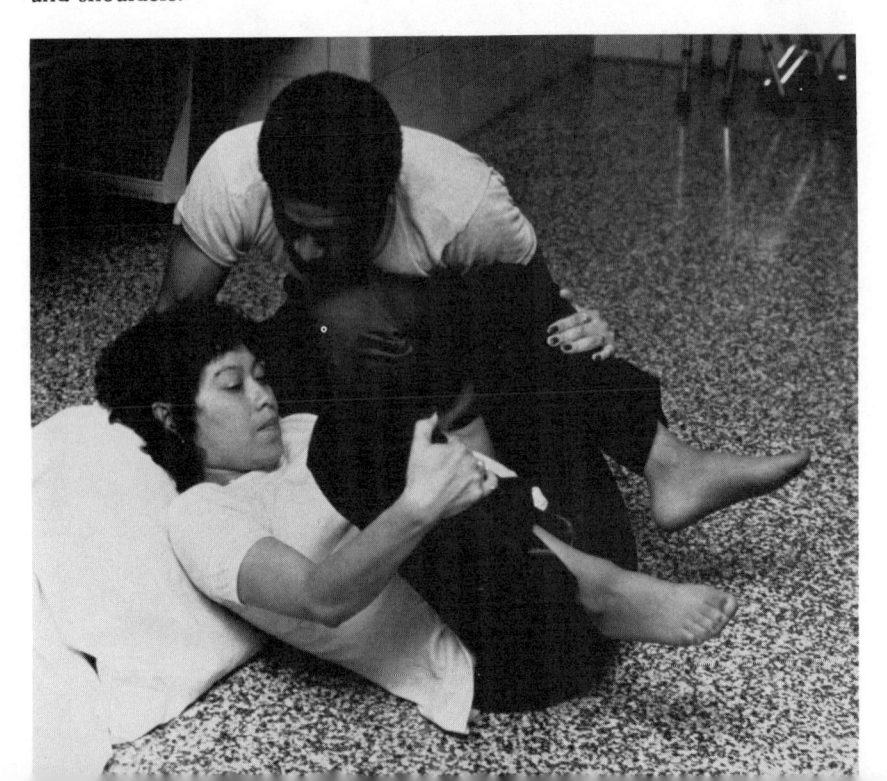

BREATHING

To push most effectively, fill your lungs with air to push your diaphragm down, bear down with your abdominal muscles, and relax the pelvic area. Since pushing is most effective at the apex of the contraction when the cervix reaches its maximum opening, take in two slow deep breaths before you begin to push. It is important that you hold your breath for as long as you can in your expelling effort so that you give your baby a smooth continual push down through the birth canal. When you can no longer hold it, exhale, take in another breath and continue pushing to the end of the contraction. You will only push during contractions. Between contractions, relax and rest as much as possible.

PATTERN

Contraction begins: Breathe in through nose, breathe out through mouth, breathe in. Breathe out.
Contraction apex: Assume your pushing position: head erect, shoulders rounded, small of back pressing against surface, pelvis tilted, buttocks and pelvic floor and legs relaxed, bearing down with abdominal muscles, pushing down and out the vaginal opening. Breathe in, hold your breath for as long as you can (practice for a count of ten to fifteen seconds), exhale slowly through pursed lips, take in another breath, and continue pushing to the end of the contraction.
Contraction ends: Finish with a cleansing breath. Lie back and relax.

Practice holding your breath for ten seconds or longer because long, controlled pushing is effective in getting your baby's head under and past the pubic bone. Think of your efforts as a slow, controlled push down and out (much as you would press your foot slowly down on the gas pedal to accelerate while driving). Short erratic breaths are counterproductive.

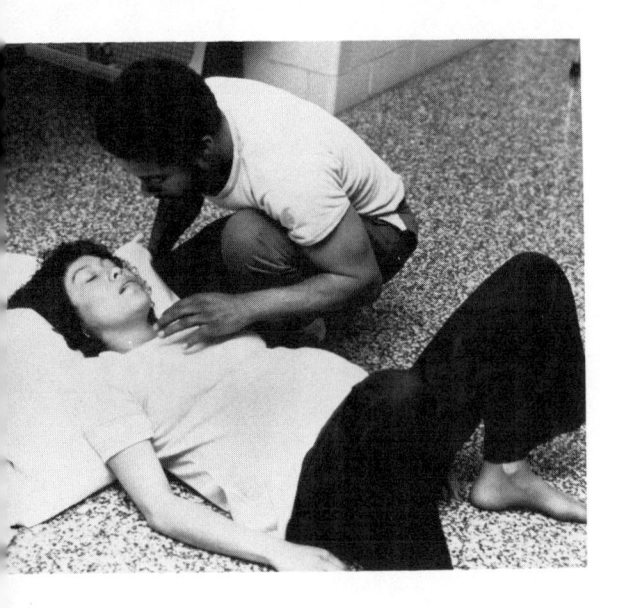

STOP PUSHING

During expulsion, as your baby moves down the birth canal through the pelvic floor, a moment will come when the largest part of his head is at the external opening. This is called the crowning. To avoid tearing the tissues of your perineum you will be asked at this time to *stop* pushing so the head may be delivered with control. Since no one can tell ahead of time exactly when the crowning will take place, you should practice responding to this command during your breathing exercises. As you are practicing your expulsion mentally verbalize your doctor's order to stop. Release your pushing position, lie back, open your mouth wide, and begin to pant in and out rapidly. This will counteract your desire to push.

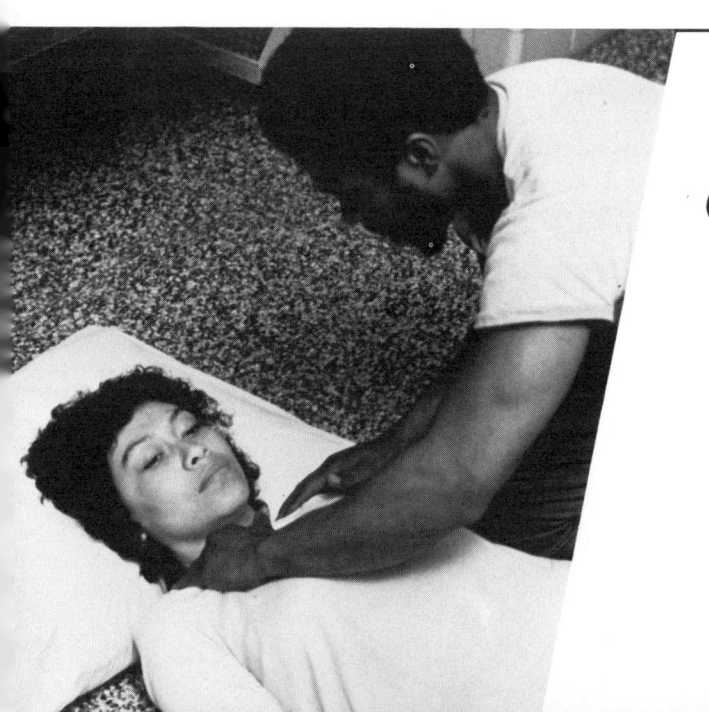

8.
Comforting Techniques

As labor progresses, it is common for the woman to experience various discomforts. An important part of childbirth preparation includes teaching both the mother and the coach ways to handle these discomforts.

PRESSURE, POSITION, AND TEMPERATURE

Much of the physical discomfort a woman may experience in labor comes from the pressure of the baby moving down through her pelvis into the birth canal. The three most effective comforting measures that you, the coach, will come armed with involve pressure, position, and temperature. These techniques are comforting for almost all women in labor.

Pressure

Massage and stroking are usually very effective during labor and delivery. Massage helps to release muscle tension, increase circulation in the muscles, and provide counterpressure to areas of discomfort. Understanding the baby's descending movement and the different points of pressure can prepare you to apply counterpressure in different areas as labor progresses.

The coach should practice all the techniques and be prepared to use or discard them as the mother's needs change. What feels good to her one moment may become uncomfortable the next. Always ask the mother what feels good, where she wants the pressure, and how much pressure she needs. Be sure she is in a comfortable position, and remind her to relax toward the massaging hands.

EFFLEURAGE

Effleurage comes from the French word that means "to skim." It implies a light stroking and may be used either by the mother or the coach during a contraction.

Using the palms and slightly cupped fingers of both hands, or only the fingertips, place them on both sides right above the pubic bone. In smooth gentle strokes they are pulled up on both sides of the uterus, come together at the top of the uterus, stroke down toward the pubic bone and, in rhythmic movement, continue in their circular paths.

The rhythm and speed should be kept steady, with the hands in constant contact with the uterus. This is usually quite effective; however, if the mother has an irritable uterus during labor, she may find it uncomfortable.

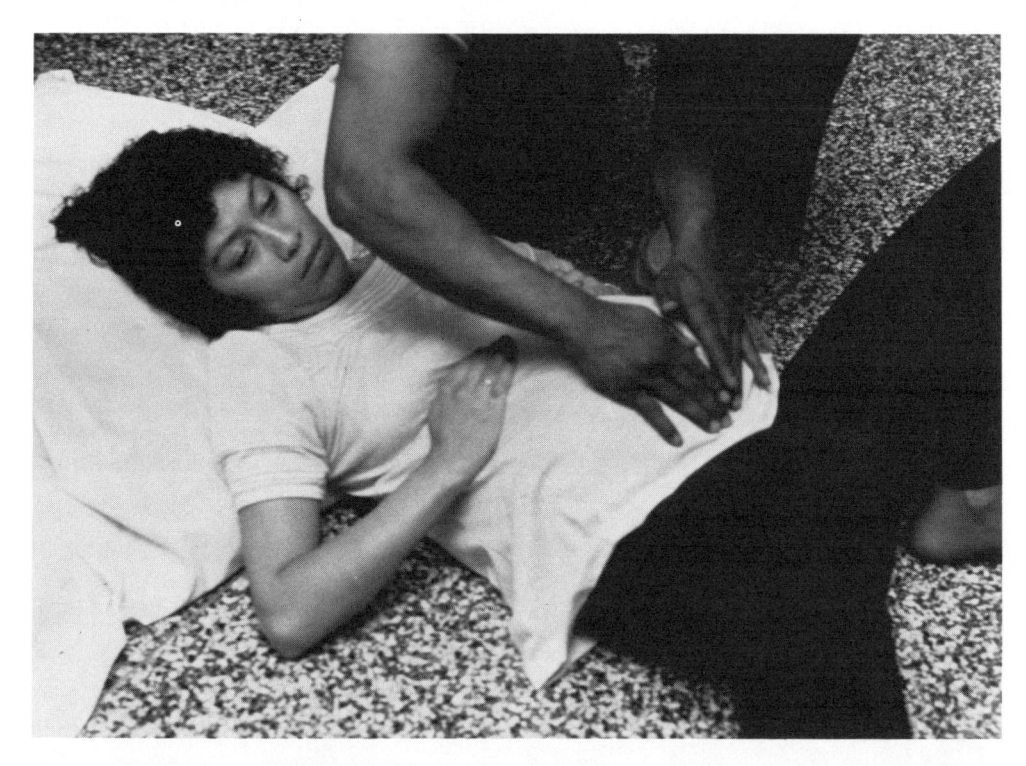

PRESSURE AREAS

Small of back. Pressure will counteract back discomforts that comes from the baby pressing on the ligaments that join the pelvis to the backbone. Pressure should be applied to the small of the mother's back with the heel of the coach's hand.

Sacrum. You can also relieve back pressure by making fists with both hands and pressing them on both sides of the mother's sacrum. She must tell you which spot feels best. Then apply steady, strong pressure in circular motions. It works best when your hand moves directly on her backbone.

Coccyx. As the baby's head descends, the mother may feel tremendous pressure and discomfort on her coccyx or lower backbone. Deep back massage and pressure against the coccyx may give her some relief. Have her lie on her side and grasp her upper hip with your hand, placing the fingers of the other hand at the beginning of the cleft between the buttocks on the tailbone. With steady pressure, stroke up about six inches toward the sacrum. The mother should press back slightly against your hands.

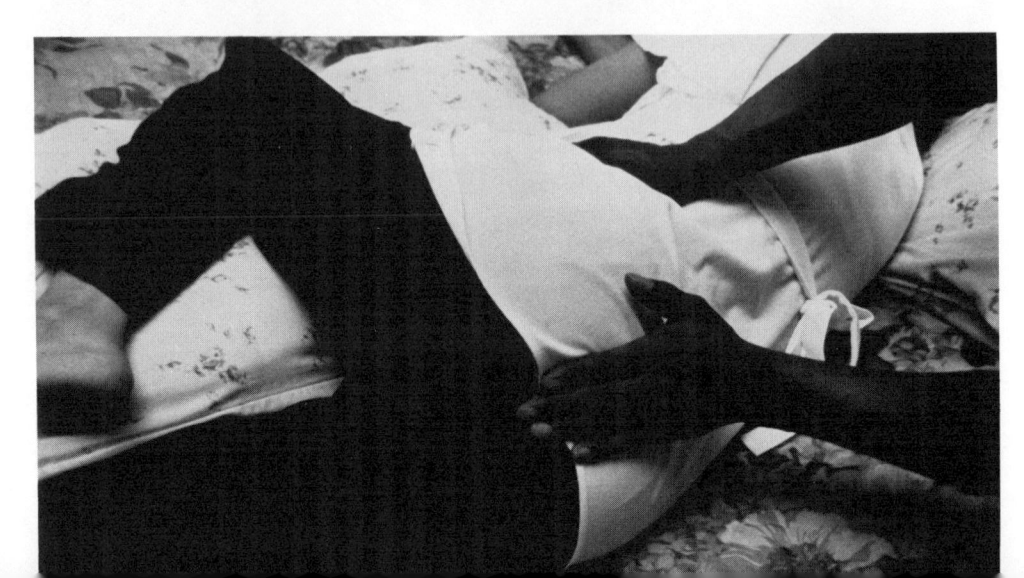

Shoulders and neck. Tense shoulder, throat, jaw, and face muscles can cause additional tension in the lower pelvic area. A firm massage about the shoulders and neck and strokes down the spinal column can help the mother relax. Remind her to keep her breathing rhythmic and unstrained, and to think of all the tension flowing out into your hands.

Buttocks and joints. The mother may feel pressure where her hipbones and legs meet. Massaging the buttocks and joints may be very helpful. The movement consists of firm massage over the buttock muscles in a slow deep movement, much like kneading bread. This is especially helpful when the baby is pressing against the mother's rectum.

Pubic bone. There may also be stress in the area under the pubic bone. Place your open palm or closed fist on the pubic bone and press with circular motions.

Pelvic floor. Toward the end of labor, the mother may feel great pressure on her pelvic floor. A strong, steady pressure on that area may give her comfort.

Position

Alternating positions can be another comforting technique for the laboring mother. To appreciate the importance that different positions have on a woman's comfort during labor, remember that in a normal labor the baby passes head first through the ischial spines, pubic bone, sacrum, and tailbone (coccyx). The joints of the pelvis have been loosened by a hormone called relaxin and are the points where the mother may feel the most pressure during labor. Side-lying and sitting positions may relieve pressure and help gravity as your baby moves.

SIDE-LYING

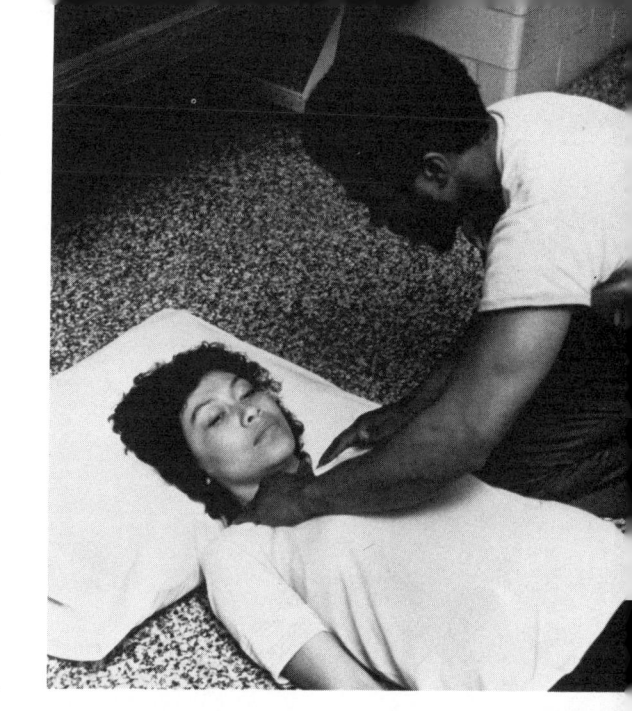

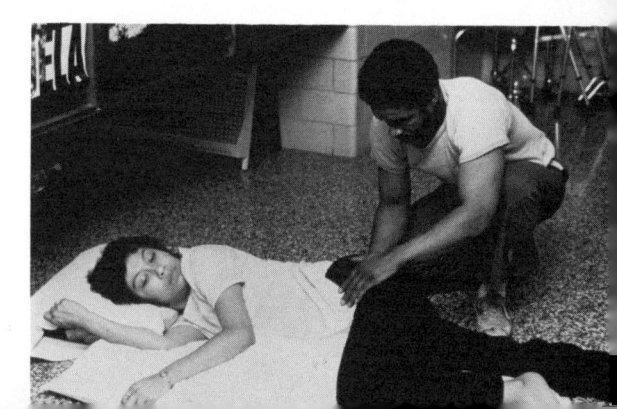

Research shows that labor in the side-lying position is more comfortable and allows more effective contractions than the supine position. The mother should lie on her side in a comfortable position. The coach should check to make sure her spine is straight and not twisted. To tilt the pelvis, the mother's upper leg should be in a bent or flexed position perpendicular to her body, with several pillows under it for support to maintain good circulation. The coach should roll a pillow and tuck it in against her back so she will have support to lean on. Pillows under her uterus or against her chest may make her more comfortable. Always be ready to change positions, since doing so makes labor more effective.

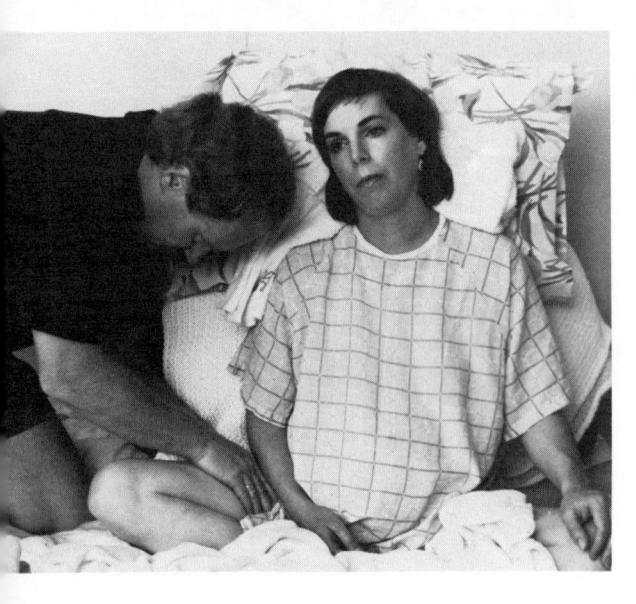

SITTING UPRIGHT

When the mother sits upright, supported by pillows, she allows gravity to help move her baby down. The coach may help her raise herself to an upright position and lean slightly forward with her legs flexed comfortably. Give her a pillow for back support and pillows under both arms. It may be comfortable to have a pillow in her lap so she can lean forward and rest her abdomen on it. Or she can lean forward using her bed table as a rest.

HANDS AND KNEES

If you, the mother, feel pressure on your back, you may want to get on your knees, buttocks in the air and elbows and forearms resting in front of you on the bed. Place your head on your arms. This removes the weight of your uterus from your back and may give relief.

Temperature

Sometimes a hot washcloth, towel, or heating pad applied to the area where the mother feels pressure helps to relieve the discomfort. If heat does not work, put ice chips in an icebag or a washcloth and towel and apply it to the area. Always remember to ask the mother what feels good and what works. Remember, again, that what was effective one moment may not work the next, and what did not work one moment may work the next.

Pure Routine

The coach can easily remember ways to comfort the mother during labor with the "PURE" memory aid.

POSITION

- Always ask the mother if she is comfortable.
- Help her avoid lying on her back, for this may impede blood and oxygen flow to the baby.
- Watch to see that her spine is straight and she is not cutting off blood to other parts of her body.
- Place pillows around her arms, legs, thighs, back, et cetera.
- Remind her to change her position every half hour.
- Be sure you yourself are in a comfortable position that is not fatiguing.

URINATION

- Remind her to urinate every hour, because the pressure on her bladder will desensitize her feelings of the need to urinate.
- Remember to urinate, yourself.

RELAXATION

- Remind her to do conscious relaxations during each contraction.
- Remind her to relax between contractions.
- Use touch and verbal commands to help her relax.
- Remind her that tension will prolong her labor.

EFFLEURAGE

- Stroke out all the tension with your hands and remind her to let all the tension flow into your hands.
- Use warm comforting hands.
- Use firm pressure; ask her what feels good, what gives the most relief.
- Remember to stroke the upper thighs; this is probably where her tension will start.
- Stroke from the main part of the body out through the extremities.
- Use rhythmical, slow stroking (do not match to pattern of breathing).
- Use soothing powder or cocoa butter to minimize trauma to the skin.

COMFORTING TOOLS TO TAKE TO THE HOSPITAL

Heat: washcloth or hot water bottle for backaches
Cold: icebag, for cramps and aches
Cornstarch or cocoa butter for massage
Chapstick, mouth spray to refresh breath
Toothbrush, toothpaste to refresh mouth
Lollipops, sour candy, tea, sugar (or honey), popsicles to refresh and give liquid
Focal point: object, picture, or photograph to concentrate on
Paper bag to breathe into in case of hyperventilation (and pack snack in for coach)
Warm socks in case feet get cold
Watch with second hand for timing contractions (if they are regular)
Books, cards, et cetera, in case you arrive at hospital in early labor
Paper and pencil to make notes and document contractions
Camera, film, flashes if you wish to take pictures
Snacks for coach: sandwiches, thermos of juice, coffee, et cetera
Coaching book

9.

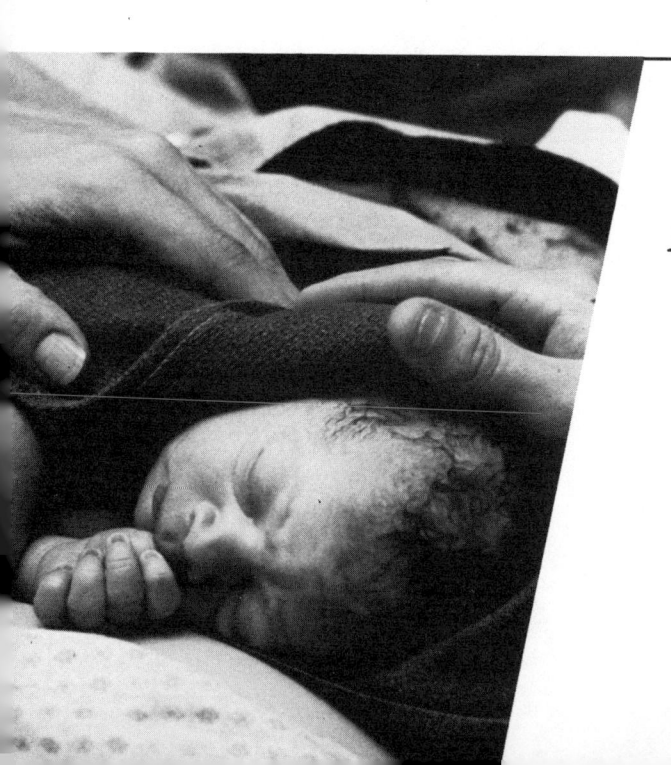

Birth

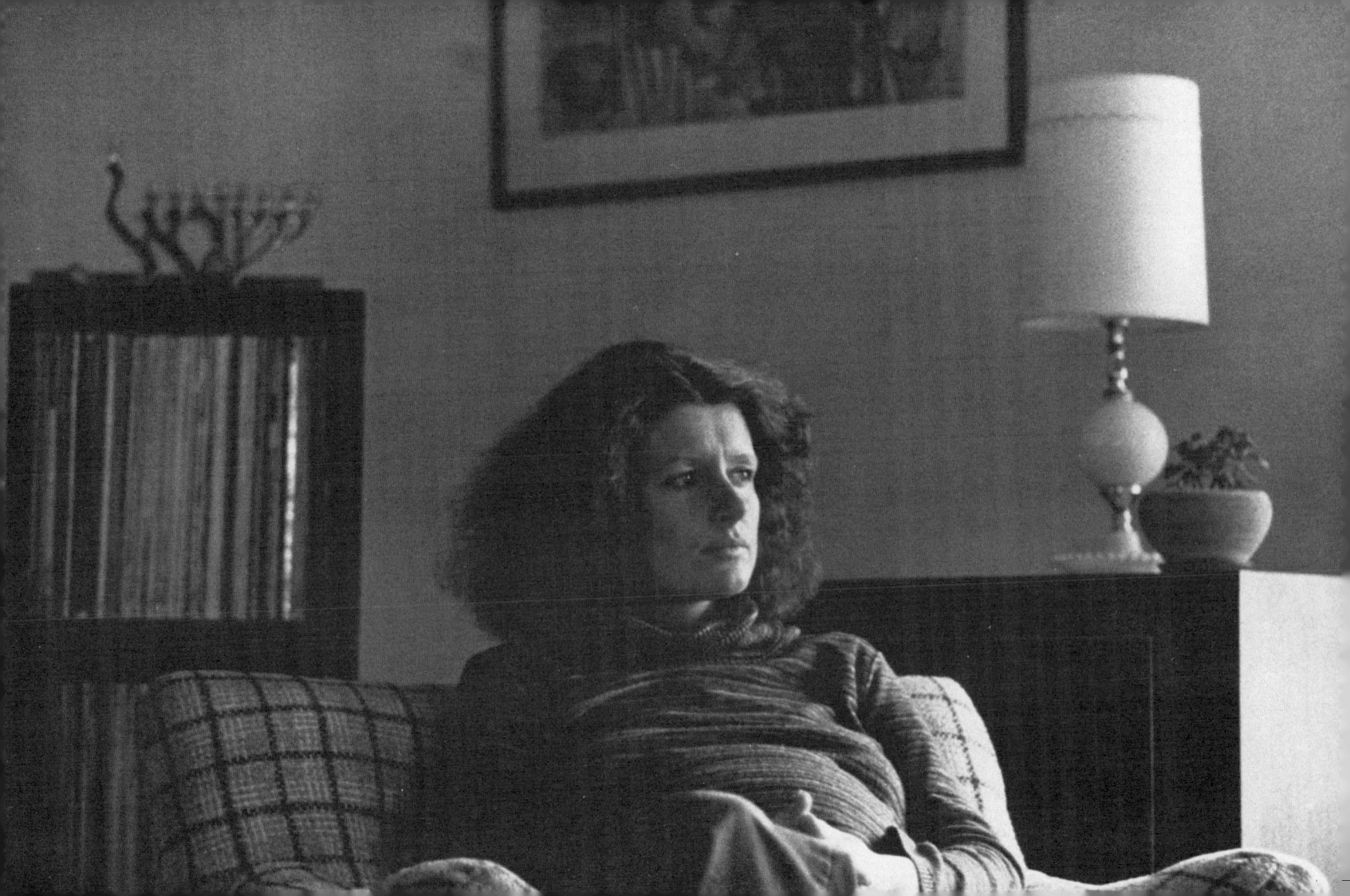

PRELABOR

During prelabor your body's systems and your baby are getting ready for the big day. Prelabor can take place two weeks, a week, or an hour before the beginning of active labor. Although no one knows what starts labor, we do know that certain physiological and hormonal events take place. Hormones in your bloodstream cause your pelvic joints to loosen in preparation for birth. They also cause the cervical tissues to soften so that they are ready to be stretched, thinned, and taken up into the uterus. At this time you might experience irregular mild contractions, felt either in your abdomen or lower back, increasing in strength and frequency.

You may experience flulike feelings, increased vaginal discharge, cramps similar to menstrual cramps, diarrhea, or a low backache. Your weight will level off or even fall. Hormones cause a mucous discharge with a pink or reddish tinge, called the "show." This is the mucous plug that sealed off the opening of your cervix during pregnancy.

You may experience what is called the "nesting urge" and want to clean the house, wash your hair, and polish the floors. It is common to have premonitions about your baby and the birth, and experience disturbing dreams that may even wake you up.

EARLY LABOR

Mother

During early labor the tissues of your cervix will be shortened and partially taken up into the body of your uterus. The opening of the cervix will begin to dilate to three or four centimeters. During the early phase, the processes of effacement and dilatation progress gradually and slowly. Your membranes may or may not rupture. If they do it is important to call your doctor or attendant.

Early labor can last 5–9 hours with your first baby and 2–5 hours with subsequent babies. Your contractions during this stage are usually mild and far apart. They may or may not be regular. They last from 15 to 45 seconds and have 10-minute to 30-minute rest intervals. They may, however, become more regular and increase in intensity. Activity increases their intensity.

POSSIBLE PHYSICAL CHANGES

You may need to urinate more frequently, feel increased pelvic pressure, and, because your digestive system is slowing down, become constipated.

POSSIBLE EMOTIONAL CHANGES

You may experience excitement and anticipation. You may also be apprehensive and anxious about the birth itself and want to talk about the coming experience with supportive friends. It is common to be anxious about whether this is true or false labor (see chapter 14). Perhaps you will be relieved that labor has finally begun. You probably feel confident that you will be able to cope with labor and birth.

WHAT TO DO

In early active labor you may wonder whether you are truly in labor or not. With your coach, assess the location of your contractions and whether they are increasing in intensity. Again, it is important that you do not dwell on your contractions (for you may go to the hospital too early if you do). Make an active effort to maintain your regular activities. Walking is a good exercise at this time. If your coach is with you, take a warm shower or bath, wash your hair, and spend time on yourself. You may want to talk to husband, friends, family, et cetera. Play cards, knit, sew, watch television, go to a movie. Eat light refreshments such as tea with honey, bouillon, fruit juices, Jello, popsicles, clear broth. Since digestion slows down with labor, don't eat hard-to-digest and complex foods such as milk. Remember to urinate every hour.

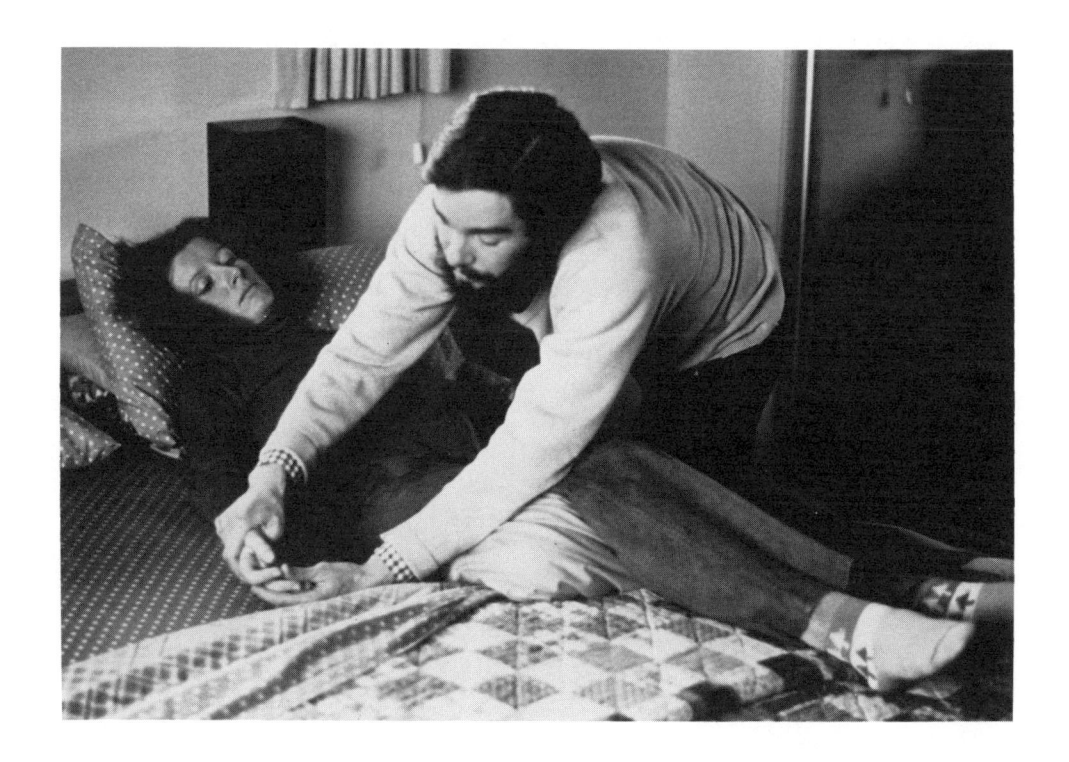

Do not go to the hospital until you experience increasingly intense contractions that you are no longer comfortable with at home. During the trip to the hospital, you may become tense and have serious doubts about labor and delivery. This is quite normal. Concentrate on your breathing, your relaxation, and listening to your coach.

Breathing. Do not begin your first-phase breathing until you can no longer easily walk, talk, or joke your way through a contraction. If you begin your active breathing too early, it ceases to be effective for the rest of the labor. When you do begin your first-phase breathing, take in a warm, relaxing cleansing breath through your nose and exhale all tension out through your mouth. Now, with easy, slow, comfortable breaths, breathe in and out throughout the contraction. End with a relaxing cleansing breath. Assess how effective the breathing is. Was it slow and quiet enough and did it feel comfortable and give you relief?

Relaxation. When you feel that you can no longer naturally relax with each contraction, begin your active relaxation with the next contraction. Concentrate on consciously releasing the tension from your toes, through your knees, thighs, pelvic floor, spine, shoulders, upper and lower arms, hands, and fingers. Relax the muscles throughout your throat and face.

Focal point. You may want to begin using your focal point at this time. Choose a point in the room that is easy to focus on and, with all your energies, concentrate on this point.

Position. During this early phase, it is helpful to constantly change your position, and to move and walk about as is comfortable to you.

Coach

At this time you are probably feeling a sense of excitement—"Yes, this may be it,"—and anxiety—"What if it isn't?" You may be asking yourself other questions, such as "What if we get to the hospital too early? What if we get to the hospital too late and I have to deliver the baby in the car?" It is common to have doubts about whether you can cope with your role as coach. You are expected to be the mother's support, and you wonder who is going to support you. On the other hand, while her contractions are not great in length, strength, or intensity, you may have feelings of great confidence in your ability to help with labor and delivery.

HOW TO HELP

During the first part of labor you are probably still at home timing the contractions, their duration, and the intervals between, and helping the mother assess when to go to the hospital. If the contractions are irregular and not growing in intensity, encourage her to conserve her energy for the oncoming labor. Reassure her about both your and her abilities to cope with the labor and delivery. Express your loving feelings and offer her moral and physical support.

COMFORTING TECHNIQUES

In this early stage your major task will be keeping the mother calm and comfortable. When you have determined that it is time to go to the hospital (or birthing site) you may wish to bring pillows or blankets. The move may be upsetting to her and if you find that she is tensing up, you may have to remind her to relax, do her deep breathing, and concentrate on a focal point with each contraction. If you have a long drive you may even want to have someone else drive so that you can coach her.

When you have finished the admission procedures and the mother is in the room where she is going to labor, your first task will probably be getting her calmed down, familiar with her room, and into a routine of dealing with her contractions. First, help her find a comfortable position. Adjust the bed and get her pillows to support her body. Find out where the bathroom is, how you get ice chips, how you call the nurse, and where you are going to change for the delivery room. You may tell the staff that you have both prepared for this childbirth, would like to be active participants, and would appreciate their support.

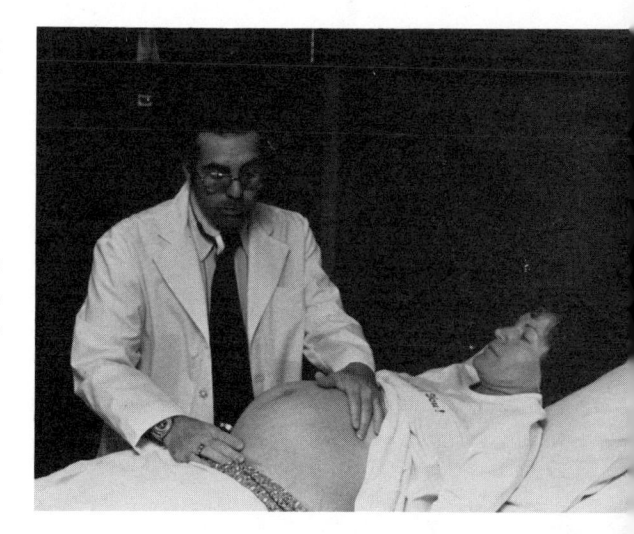

ACTIVE LABOR

Mother

During the active phase of labor, your contractions become more intense because they are doing more work. Your cervix is completely effaced and is dilating to 7 cm. Your baby's presenting part (usually the head) is moving downward into your bony pelvis. During this active phase, dilatation progresses more rapidly. If your membranes have ruptured or rupture during this phase, you can expect progress to be further hastened. This period usually lasts from three to six hours with your first baby and half as long with subsequent births.

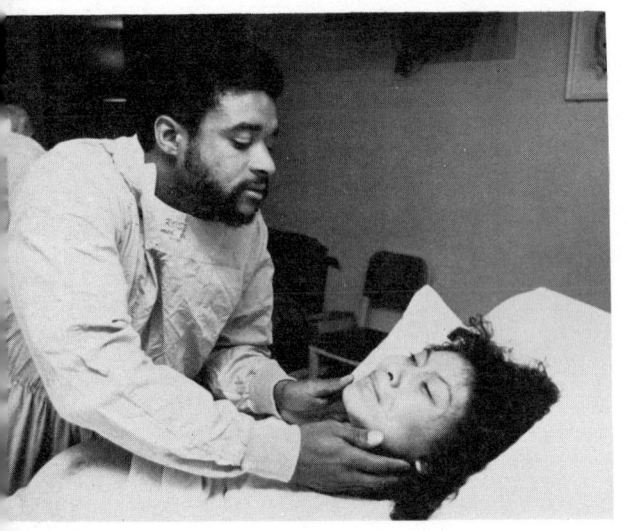

POSSIBLE PHYSICAL CHANGES

When you arrive at the hospital, you may experience an alteration in the pattern of your contractions. They may slow down, become irregular or even stop for a short time. As your labor progresses you will notice a gradual increase in your bloody show. You may begin to experience discomfort in your back, hips, and legs with cramping in your feet or thighs.

POSSIBLE EMOTIONAL CHANGES

As the intensity of the contractions mounts and labor continues, you usually get more serious about your labor. You may become quiet and preoccupied with your work, and you may not wish to keep up a conversation. As your contractions mount you have to use greater concentration to remain in control. You may resent distractions and have a feeling of panic or "no return." You may begin to doubt your ability to cope with the stress of labor and birth. You may fear that you can't do it without the support of your coach, doctor, nurse, and medical staff.

WHAT TO DO

In this period of active labor, it is your job to catch each contraction as it starts and work with it through its apex to the end. You must concentrate on taking advantage of the rest period between contractions. Listen to your coach: help him to assess each contraction's location, beginning, peak, and ending, and the rest period in between. Concentrating on your breathing, relaxation, focal point, and coach's stroking and voice will help distract your attention from the intensity of your contractions. Remember to empty your bladder every hour.

Breathing. When deep slow breathing no longer works for you (i.e., meets the intensity of the contractions and helps you stay in control), it is time to switch to the shallow accelerated type of breathing at the peak of each contraction. Pick a focal point and use your cleansing breath as a signal to your coach that a contraction is beginning and ending. Then use your slow deep breathing as long as you can, switch to the accelerated breathing when you need it, and go back to slow chest breathing as the contraction lets up. No matter what the pattern of the contraction (early peak, piggyback, et cetera), match the highest intensity with accelerated breathing and the lower intensity with deep slow breathing. If the accelerated breathing does not work for you, be sure to go back to your deep slow breathing. Should you feel any tingling in your fingers, toes, or nose, tell your coach as soon as possible so that he may take steps to keep you from hyperventilating.

Relaxation. As your contractions mount in intensity it will take even more concentration to control your relaxation. Listen to your coach; concentrate on his voice and touch. When your coach begins his stroking, concentrate on releasing all the tension in your body out through his hands.

It is important that you tell your coach not only where you feel pressure and aches (remember, they will change as your baby moves down), but also which techniques give you the greatest comfort. Tell him if you want the pressure softer or harder; if you want his hands farther up or down; if you want heat or cold; and tell him when it feels good. Tell him if your position is comfortable or uncomfortable. Ask for pillows, support, ice chips, fluids as you need them.

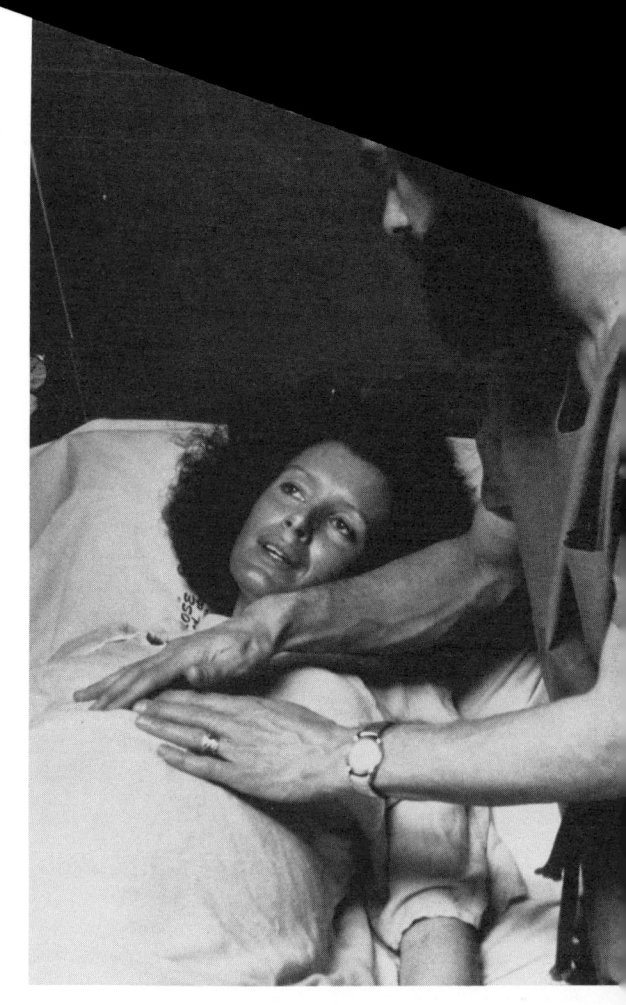

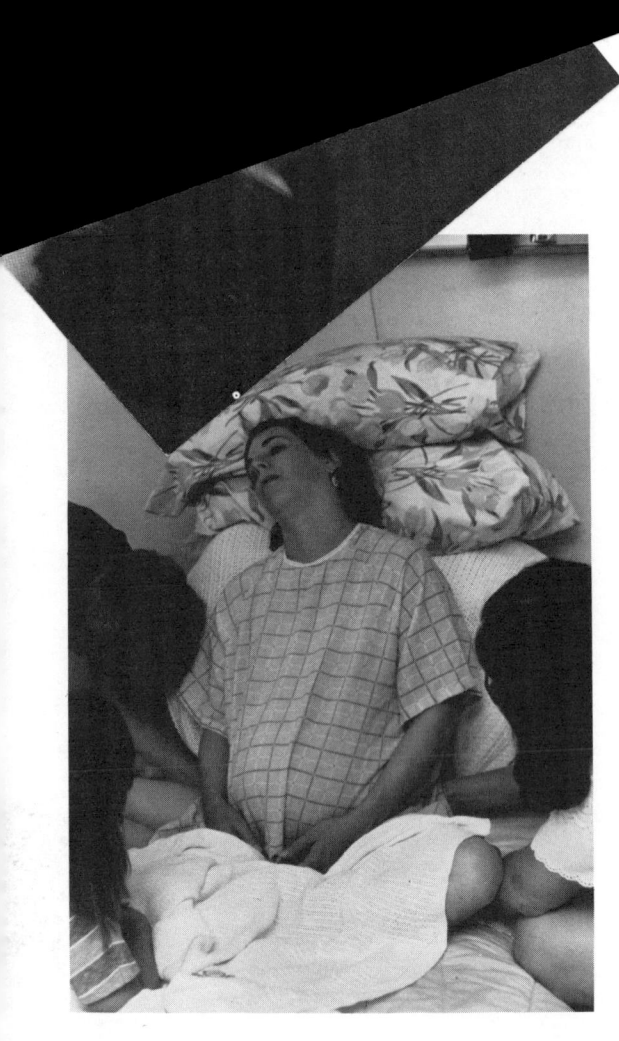

Position. Remember to change your position every thirty minutes. You may not want to walk around at this stage, but if you do, it may help your labor. The side-lying position has been shown to be not only more comfortable (baby off spine), but to result in more effective contractions. If you have a backache, try rocking on all fours. You may want to stand and lean over your bed table. If you do lie on your back, assume a semi-sitting position so you are not putting pressure on the blood vessels that bring oxygen to your baby.

Coach

As labor progresses, you may begin to realize the necessity for a great deal of effort on your part. By now, however, you have established a pattern. Each time a contraction starts it is the mother's signal to begin her breathing, relaxation, focal point, and concentration techniques and your signal to begin your comforting, instruction, and encouragement. You are working hard but you realize the importance of your role because of the obvious support and relief you are giving the laboring mother.

HOW TO HELP

Analyze the contractions: where do they start, when do they reach their apex, when do they let off? Where does the mother feel them (front, back, et cetera)? Find out if the contractions are regular and, if they are, timing will probably be very helpful during labor. If the contractions are irregular, timing may be discouraging. Continue to monitor the contractions and their changing qualities as they become longer, stronger, and closer together. Keep the mother informed about the progress of her labor after each examination. As her labor progresses she will probably be surprised by the growing intensity of her contractions and sensations of discomfort. Reassure her that these sensations are normal and her labor is progressing as it should.

COMFORTING TECHNIQUES

Encourage her to find a comfortable position and to change her position every thirty minutes. Adjust pillows under her head, uterus, back, legs, and arms to give her support. Experiment with massaging her sacrum, coccyx, hipbones, and pubic bone until you find where pressure gives her the most relief. Be sure to put cornstarch or cocoa butter on the skin you are touching. Be prepared to change massage techniques as the baby moves down. Use heat and cold on pressure points. A cool cloth may feel good on her forehead. Ask her if she wants ice chips. She may enjoy a lollipop or tea with sugar or honey for energy. Chapstick on her lips, or brushing her teeth between contractions, may refresh her mouth. Remind her to empty her bladder every hour. Be sure to keep up your energy with snacks and empty your bladder when you need to. Toward the end of this stage, you may want to dress for delivery so you will not have to leave her during transition.

TRANSITION

Mother

Until now, your contractions have caused the thinning out and dilatation of your cervix. Now, you will notice a difference both in the quality and intensity of the contractions and in the sensations and pressure you will feel. Your contractions will begin their preparations for expelling the baby, and the areas in which you feel pressure will change as he moves down through your pelvis into your birth canal. Although this is the most difficult period in your labor, it is also the shortest. Transition may last anywhere from ten minutes to one hour.

CONTRACTIONS

Your contractions will not only become extremely strong, but they will often be erratic. They will last 60–90 seconds with only short rest periods in between. Their quality changes in that they not only peak quickly, but they may piggyback on one another, giving you little or no time to rest. This, along with constant pressure on the pelvic floor, may give you the feeling that they never end.

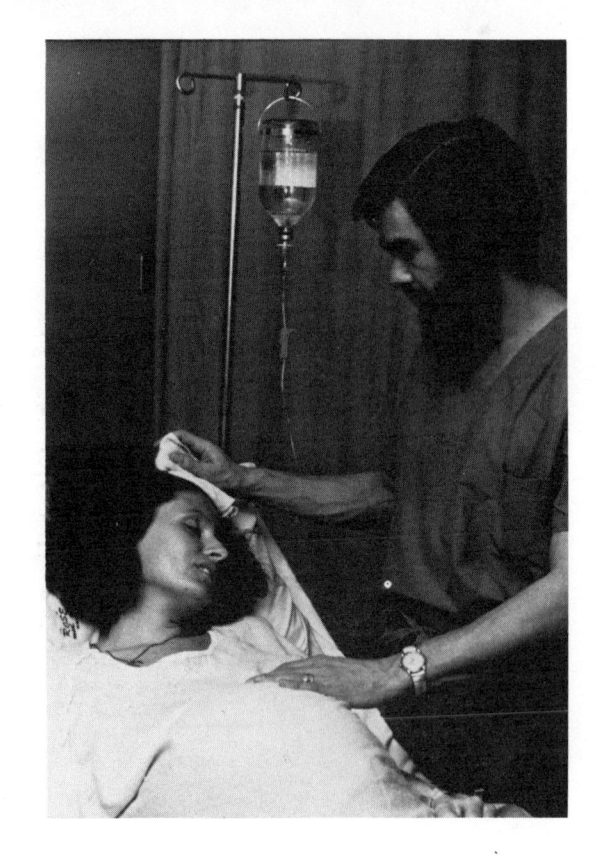

POSSIBLE PHYSICAL CHANGES

Probably the most striking sign of transition is a sudden and overwhelming desire to bear down with your abdominal muscles, even though your cervix is not completely dilated. Although not all women experience this, the majority do. As your baby moves down through your pelvis into the birth canal you may feel intense pressure on your pelvic floor and pressure in your rectum almost as if you are going to have a bowel movement. This may be accompanied by a dark, heavy mucous discharge. Hot flashes, red blotchy cheeks, and perspiration appearing on your forehead and upper lip, mixed intermittently with chills and shivering, are familiar signs of transition. You may experience cold feet as your baby moves down and slows your circulation. Some women get an overwhelming desire to go to sleep and escape. Some experience low back pain, burping, hiccoughs, nausea, vomiting, and trembling during transition.

POSSIBLE EMOTIONAL CHANGES

This period is the most intense physically and emotionally. You will probably experience your most extreme feelings and sensations, and maybe even undergo a temporary personality change. The change may sneak up on you slowly, or it may hit you suddenly. As the uterus uses more and more oxygen, there is a poorer supply of oxygen to your brain and it is common to experience an overwhelming feeling that you can't stay in control of your contractions. Beginning with feelings of restlessness and irritability, you may become panicky, discouraged, fatigued, and confused. You may forget how to do your breathing patterns and how to relax to your coach's commands. You may feel trapped and wish to escape from your body, your labor, and the birth. You may even want to go home. You are frightened at being left alone, and may panic if your coach leaves for any reason. You may turn inward and forget concerns about modesty and the impression you are making on others.

WHAT TO DO

The physical and emotional changes that occur during the transitional stage may sound frightening, but you are unlikely to experience all of these sensations all of the time. Some women experience none of the transitional phase as described. Others experience only a few of the sensations. What is important is that you and your coach go into labor armed with techniques to counteract these discomforts.

Transition will probably be the hardest work you have ever done in your life. The most helpful thing you can do during this phase is to respond to your coach with all your concentration and all your determination. Let him guide you. Listen to his instructions, his encouragement, and his support.

Things to remember:

- *This is the shortest stage,* and your baby will soon arrive.
- *Don't give up; you are not alone.* Your coach is with you and will help you. He will get you through one contraction at a time.
- *Don't panic.* The intensity of the contraction is overwhelming, but nothing is wrong. They are natural and normal and an important part in the process of birth.
- *Tension will prolong transition* (which is good for neither you nor your baby). If you get out of control you must concentrate with all your power on your coach's directions, his voice, and his touch. He can get you back in control only if you cooperate and let him.

Breathing. When the contraction begins, concentrate on your focal point. As the contraction becomes stronger and your desire to push appears, you will find that the transitional breathing techniques of short breaths mixed with pants will give you relief. Be sure to start your transition breathing pattern as soon as you feel your contraction begin. As your contractions mount in intensity, decrease the pants and increase the blows. When the desire to push becomes overwhelming, give several blows at the peak of the contraction to help counteract the desire to push. If you get out of control look at your coach to help you.

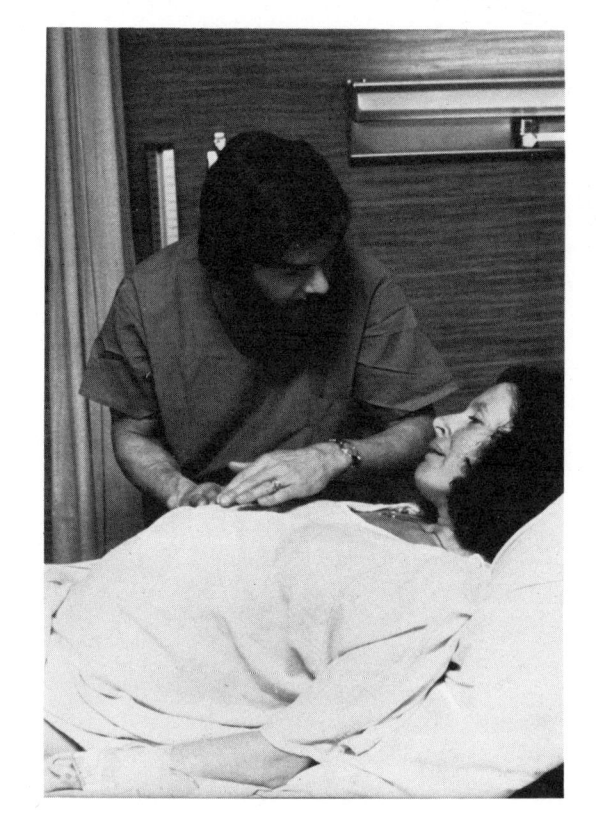

Relaxation. Probably the most difficult task will be relaxing. You will feel tremendous pressure in your pelvis as your baby moves down and tremendous pressure in the birth canal, as well as a new sensation as your abdominal muscles begin to bear down involuntarily. It will take an extra effort to relax, but concentrate on your coach's directions and his touch. Remind yourself that if you tense up you will prolong your labor, and if you relax you will shorten this stage. Concentrate on releasing the tension in your pelvic floor and thighs. Relax your face and shoulders. As your baby moves down and you feel pressure areas change, tell your coach so he can change his massage and comfort pressures. Express your needs for massage, heat, cold, and fluids.

Position. Find the position that is most comfortable to you. Ask your coach for pillows to support all of your body so you can relax into them. Try the side-lying position so your coach can massage your back. If you have a backache, try the all-fours position.

Coach

It is not unusual for the first-time coach to feel overwhelmed by the intensity of transition just as the mother does. You may think something has gone wrong and become anxious. Don't panic; be assured that not only is it normal but, for the practiced coach, transition is exciting because it means that labor is almost over and it will not be long before the birth of your baby. Your major job will be remaining calm and in control for both the mother who is laboring and for you, who by this time is also laboring.

If you are going to change into delivery room clothes, do it at the earliest signs of transition (if not before). The laboring woman needs your continual encouragement, support, and comforting. She is lost if you leave her even to go to the bathroom.

HOW TO HELP

Transition is the time the laboring woman needs your coaching the most. Your encouragement, praise, support, and instruction take on even more importance for her. Transition is your time to take over. You must be firm and direct and take charge of her relaxation, breathing, and control. Since she may become confused, you must be sure that all of your instructions are given in a firm reassuring tone and in simple, clear language. Increase your eye contact and your verbal and touching support measures to help her most effectively.

Remind the mother that although this may be the most difficult time, it also means that the birth is not far away. Remind her firmly that if she listens to your directions, you will help her through each contraction, and that if she allows herself to tense and get out of control, she will only prolong her labor.

You will take one contraction at a time. With each contraction you will help her monitor her breathing and relaxation techniques and will give her relief with your comforting techniques. It will be your job to alert the mother at the beginning of each contraction to help her begin her breathing techniques and to help her with the increasingly difficult task of remaining relaxed and in control. *If she becomes irritable and frustrated, don't take it as a personal insult.* Think of it as a physiological condition in which the uterus is using so much oxygen it is impossible for her to function as usual. Try to remain calm and understanding.

COMFORTING TECHNIQUES

Now you are really busy with your comforting techniques. She may need everything you have in your bag of tricks plus more. You will need to expect that some of the things you have practiced may not give her any relief and, indeed, may increase her discomfort. You must be prepared to abandon these measures and proceed with others that do give her relief. If you think of something that might help her that hasn't been mentioned, try it.

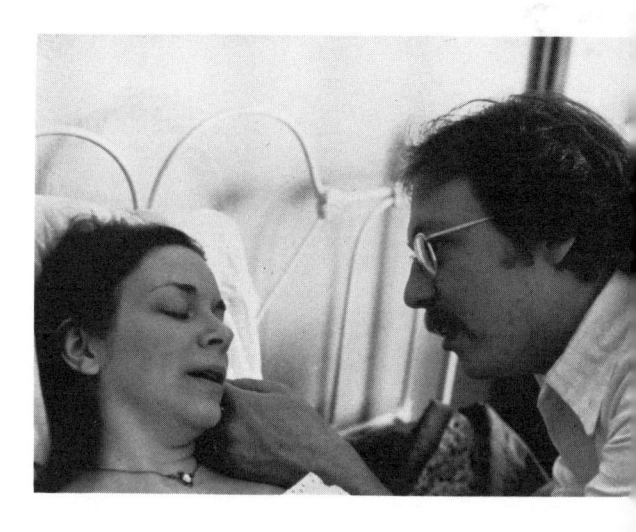

Massage and pressure. You can probably expect her to feel some sort of back discomfort, so be prepared to use your massage techniques. Turning her on her side and using either your fists or palms of both hands, try massaging both sides of the sacrum. Be sure to ask her where the pressure gives her the most relief. As the baby moves down, try firm pressure on the coccyx. She may prefer one fist right in the middle of the sacrum. If she feels discomfort in her hipbones, massage in a kneading manner where the hipbone goes into the pelvis. If she feels discomfort in her buttocks, knead the buttocks area. Some women feel discomfort in the front where the pelvis comes together at the pubic bone. Using the palm on your hand, exert pressure right on the pubic bone. As the baby moves down even further and the mother feels pressure on the rectal area, place the palm of your hand directly on the rectal area on the pelvic floor and press up; this may give her great relief.

In between contractions, massage and stroke her face, neck, shoulders, and spine to help her relax these areas.

Heat and cold. Heat and cold may give her great relief at this time. On all of the pressure areas just discussed (sacrum, coccyx, hipbones, buttocks, pubic bone, et cetera), try placing a cloth or towel soaked in hot water to see if it gives her comfort. If not, try placing cloths soaked in cold water on these areas.

OTHER POSSIBLE PROBLEMS

Other discomforts she may experience that you should be prepared for are: cold feet, hot flashes, leg cramps, rectal pressure, trembling, shivering, nausea, sleepiness, confusion, irritability, and loss of control.

Hot and cold. It is common for the mother to experience both hot and cold. She will feel hot from all the energy she is expending. Her face may be flushed and perspiring. A cold, wet washcloth on her forehead and face may feel especially good.

At the same time her feet may be cold. Because her uterine muscles are consuming so much oxygen, the circulation to her feet may be impaired. A pair of wool socks will feel good.

Leg cramps. Sometimes a woman may experience painful leg cramps. To prevent them, be sure to remove any restrictive clothing (such as tight socks). Stroke her groin, thighs, and legs between contractions and remind her to relax her legs. Tell her to think of them as butter melting into the bed. Should she experience a cramp during contractions, have her extend her leg straight out; then, grasping her heel in one hand and her toes in the other, pull on her heel and push her toes toward her knees. Remind her to relax as much as possible. She can also experience relief by pushing her foot against your hands or chest.

Rectal pressure. The mother may experience extreme rectal pressure and think she has to have a bowel movement. In fact, it is very common for the contractions to feel more comfortable while she is sitting on the toilet. This is because squatting is the normal pushing position. Remind her to keep her perineum as relaxed as possible, since tension will slow her labor and cause pain.

Trembling, shivering. Shivering or trembling in the mother's lower limbs may be a reaction to increased exertion of the uterus. It may also occur when her membranes rupture. Have the mother take a deep breath and hold it for five seconds, releasing it as slowly as possible. Repeat several times. Sometimes holding her legs firmly eases the trembling.

Nausea, vomiting. When the mother goes into active labor, activity in her digestive system comes to a stop, and as her labor progresses she may experience nausea or even vomiting caused by sensitivity and tension in the diaphragm. It is not uncommon to burp or vomit during transition. If she feels nauseated, tell her to take a breath and let it escape slowly through her lips, concentrating on relaxing her whole body.

Sleepiness. During transition is is common for the laboring woman to become sleepy, either because she has been awake a long time or because of the increased concentration needed during the birth process. Because of the tremendous consumption of oxygen and the brain's resultant oxygen deprivation, the mother commonly experiences amnesia during the transitional phase of labor. Allowing the mother to sleep between contractions may help her to replenish her energy, but the coach should make sure to wake her before the next contraction so she may meet it with her relaxation and breathing techniques.

Confusion. When the uterus uses so much oxygen and the brain is deprived, the mother may find it difficult to concentrate and become confused. This is why preparation and conditioned response are so important.

You may find it helpful to count the mother's breathing patterns out loud for her, or even breathe with her. Remember to use the rate and pattern that is right for her, not your own. Remind her to keep it as slow, even, and comfortable as possible. As she tunes in to you, keep the outside distraction and jokes to a minimum. Try to give her a fifteen-second warning before the contraction begins and give her plenty of encouragement. Assure her that she is not alone. Remind her to concentrate on her relaxation, her breathing, her focal point, and on the stroking of your hands taking away the tension.

Irritability. Oxygen deprivation may also result in irritability. When a woman becomes irritable, it is a good sign that she is in transition and that her labor is almost over. You must try to be understanding and patient. Remind her that transition is usually short and that the birth of the baby is not far away. The nurse and doctor are probably there and will even be guessing the time of the arrival of your newborn. It may help the mother to have her dilatation checked, because at this time, things usually begin to move quickly and knowledge of her progress is encouraging.

Loss of control. What does "losing control" mean? The mother may begin to tense up her arms and legs as if she were going to roll into a ball when the contraction starts. She may grip your hand and begin to toss from side to side. In the middle of the contraction she will stop her breathing techniques and say that she cannot (or will not) continue with her relaxation or breathing. You may hear her say things that you know she would never normally say. All this is not unusual, and is an indication that transition is almost over. However, since tension and loss of control will prolong this stage and make birth even more difficult, it is important that you pick up these signals early and deal firmly with her to get her back into control.

Recognize the signs of getting out of control and act to get her into control as soon as possible. The longer you let it go, the harder it will be. First try to help her get through the contraction that she has lost control of and then, in the rest interval, tell her that she is not alone, that you are going to work with her, one contraction at a time, so that she will remain in control, but that she must listen to your directions and respond to them. Tell her that transition is the sign that the baby is almost there and that if she loses control now, she will only prolong the transition stage for both herself and her baby.

The three key methods that will help you get her back into control are eye contact, firm voice, and a secure touch. You must first get her to open her eyes and look at you. You may have to be firm to get through to her at this time. Say distinctly and firmly:

"Mary, open your eyes and look at me." You may have to grasp her face with both hands and bring your face down close to hers. Continue saying "Open your eyes and look at me," again and again, until she does so. It may take several times. Remind her that it is to her advantage to open her eyes and look at you because tension will only prolong labor. This in itself may be very effective because no woman wants to prolong her transition.

If she tries to shut her eyes tighter, or wiggle out of your hands, keep your hands firmly on her face, call her name, and repeat "Open your eyes and look at me." Continue until she opens her eyes and looks directly into your eyes. Tell her "I'm going to help you."

When her eyes are open, you can begin to work on her breathing. Again, with a firm voice and both hands on her face, say "Open your mouth," (she has probably forgotten how to breathe). Once her mouth is open tell her "Now breathe in; now breathe out." Again, she may not hear you and you must tell her several times. As you get her breathing in and out deeply, you will feel her body gradually beginning to relax. Keeping her breathing steady, move your hands down to her shoulders and begin to stroke them, reminding her to keep her eyes open, her breathing steady. As you stroke her arms and legs, tell her to relax to the touch of your hands. Tell her she is not alone, that you are with her all the way. Tell her that you will help her through each contraction, and that you will take only one contraction at a time. You will finally begin to feel her get back into control. Continue to give her support, instructions, directions, and encouragement. She will never need it more, nor will the rewards be greater. Keep emphasizing she is not alone and the two of you can do it together.

Many women with their first babies become so overwhelmed by transition that they forget it is only a temporary period and begin to fear that the intensity will never stop mounting. It is usually at this time that even the most fervent antimedication mother begins to think that maybe anesthesia (or even a cesarean!) doesn't sound too bad. However, before she chooses to take anything, remind her that transition is usually only a short period. With the help of her birthing attendant, evaluate how long she has been in labor and how quickly the cervix is dilating. If she has been in labor for only a short time to average time and the cervix is dilating smoothly, you can tell her that the birth is close.

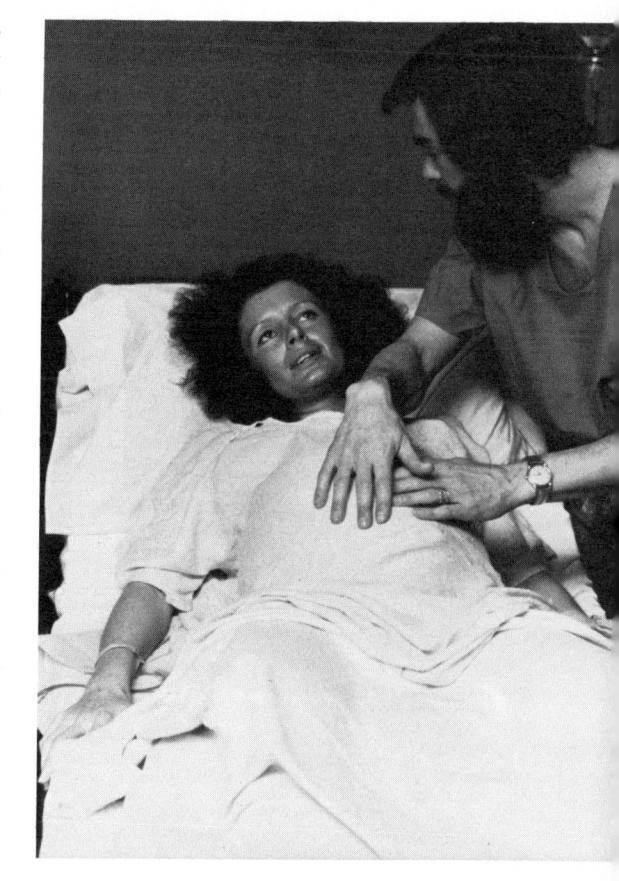

If her labor has been very long and the cervix is dilating quite slowly, she may find transition unendurable. If she is fatigued, her pain level will be quite low and the rest induced by medication may actually shorten labor. It is important to discuss medications with your birthing attendant before labor begins. Know what may be given, and what the side effects are for both the mother and the baby. Remember, the health of your baby is the first priority. If you have chosen a physician who is in tune with your philosophy, and who does not use anesthesia as a routine procedure, you can feel quite confident in his or her advice.

DELIVERY

Mother

When your cervix has dilated to 10 centimeters, your baby is ready to pass through your vagina. As he descends through the birth canal, his head rests on the floor of your pelvic region. If the membranes of the amniotic sac have not ruptured earlier in birth, a gush of fluid from your vagina occurs during expulsion. Now, in addition to the involuntary contractions of the uterus, it is time to bear down with your abdominal muscles, directing all your energy toward pushing your baby out.

As the vagina begins to open you can see your baby for the first time. With each contraction, the perineum bulges more and more, and the opening to the vagina becomes distended by your baby's head, so that it gradually changes from a small slit to a circle. As each contraction stops, the head recedes and the opening becomes smaller. With the next contraction, the opening enlarges more.

As the head becomes visible, the vagina is stretched further and finally encircles the largest diameter of your baby's head. This is called the crowning. The doctor asks you to stop pushing, so that you do not tear the perineum, and your baby's head emerges between contractions. Once the head appears, your baby takes a first breath. Since some babies swallow mucus coming down the birth canal, the doctor may use suction to clear your baby's airway.

Almost immediately after your baby's head turns to the side, the shoulders are born. The upper shoulder appears under the pubic arch and stops temporarily, acting as a pivot point for the other shoulder. As the upper part of the perineum becomes distended, the other shoulder emerges. The pushing and delivery phase lasts from fifteen minutes to two hours.

CONTRACTIONS

Contractions during this stage are powerful, but they have a different and more manageable quality than those of transition. They last 60–90 seconds with intervals 1–3 minutes in between. They are shorter, less intense, and have a longer rest phase. But, most important, the mother's perception of the contractions changes because she is an active participant and is pushing out her baby.

POSSIBLE PHYSICAL CHANGES

As your baby's head moves farther down, you may experience great rectal and perineal pressure. You may experience increased amnesia between your contractions. With the gradual appearance of your baby's presenting part at your vaginal opening you may experience a stretching, tearing, or burning sensation at the perineum and even a feeling of "splitting open." During the contractions, you may grunt involuntarily.

Since circulation of the blood to the perineal area is restricted, your legs may shake. The pressure of your baby's head against the nerves of the birth canal may numb the canal until after the birth is complete. If an episiotomy is done, you will probably not feel it.

POSSIBLE EMOTIONAL CHANGES

When you start to push, you will start to feel less muddled and confused. As you take a more active role in labor, you begin to experience a decrease in pain and your determination and energy begin to return.

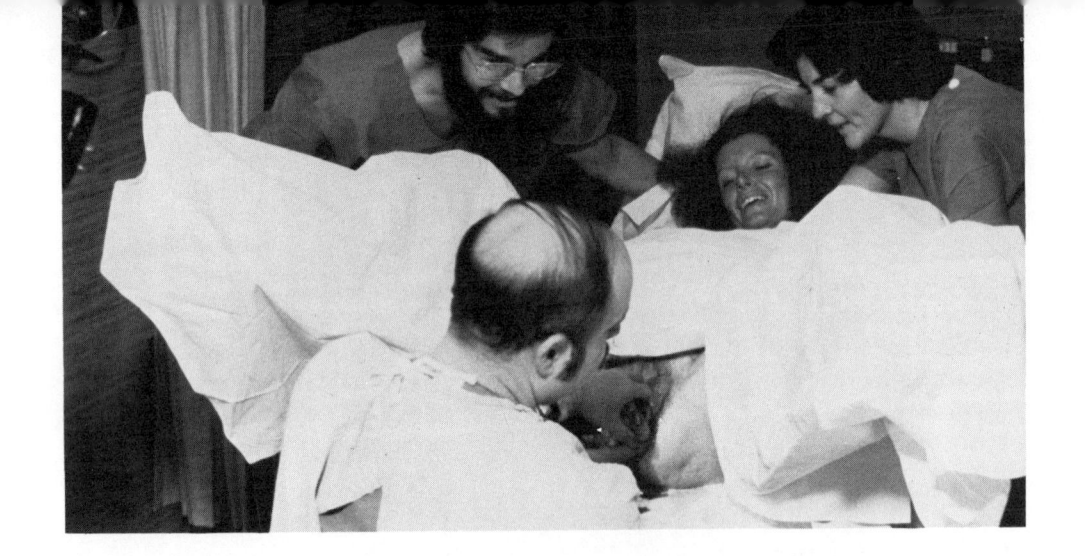

You may feel an excitement and exhilaration about your baby being born. You become increasingly involved in the birth process and experience tremendous satisfaction with each push. On the other hand, some women feel acute pain with each push and, as they get to the end of the delivery, they feel completely exhausted after each contraction. If you have a long labor you may be unable to follow the attendant's directions readily and will have to look to your coach.

When the baby's head is finally delivered you may experience feelings of relief. When your baby's body is delivered you may feel joy, awe, surprise, and fear. You will be concerned about your body and need assuring that you did indeed survive the experience.

WHAT TO DO

It is important during this phase that you do not push until you are told that the cervix is completely dilated, because pushing on the incompletely dilated cervix may be painful. When the signal comes to push, remember: position, breathing, relaxation, and control.

Position. First, choose a pushing position that is comfortable. Be sure your pelvis is tilted, your perineum relaxed, legs spread on both sides of the uterus, small of the back straight, shoulders rounded, arms bent and out, neck straight, and head erect (not down on your chest). If you are in the delivery room be sure to tell the attendant if your legs and arms are uncomfortable or if you cannot see in the mirror.

Breathing. As the contraction starts, take in a slow breath, exhale, take in another slow breath, exhale; then, take in another slow breath (this will get you to the peak of the contraction), hold your breath, and with a controlled effort, bear down with your abdominal muscles. Your coach will count for you. Hold your breath as long as you can (or, for a variation, slowly let out your breath through pursed lips). Concentrate on pushing your baby down and out the vaginal canal with a strong, steady, sustaining effort. Think "down and out." When you need to take another breath, keep your pushing position so that you retain the position of your baby's head and let out the breath you have been holding. Take in another deep breath and continue pushing to the end of the contraction.

Do not hold back your pushing efforts because you feel you are going to have a bowel movement; you aren't. When, at the crowning, your birthing attendant tells you to stop pushing, release your pushing position, open your mouth, and begin to pant. Some women experience an exhilarating burst of sensation much like an orgasm at the moment of birth.

Relaxation. While you are pushing, relax your thighs and calves and concentrate on relaxing your pelvic floor and your perineum. It helps to concentrate also on relaxing your face and mouth. When the contraction is over, it is important that you lie back and relax as much as possible to recover your energy for the next contraction.

Coach

Excitement now becomes a part of the scene. You are relieved to see that the mother has gotten an extra supply of energy, has lost her confused and irritable state, and is herself becoming excited about the birth of the baby. Depending on the length and intensity of the labor, and how hard you had to work, your feelings will vary from relief to great joy.

HOW TO HELP

With the first push help her get into a comfortable position with her back curved, pelvis tilted, shoulders rounded, and arms out. Point out the abdominal muscles with which she will be bearing down and remind her to concentrate on relaxing her toes, feet, thighs, and perineum.

COMFORTING TECHNIQUES

If the mother is to be moved to the delivery room, be sure that they move her between contractions. The move may be difficult for her. Try to stay by her and, as she experiences a contraction, help her with her breathing and relaxation.

Remember to bring pillows in with you. If she is going to use the leg supports on the delivery table, see that they are comfortably positioned for her. If she is going to use a mirror to see the birth, be sure it is in position. If she does not wish to use wristcuffs, tell the attendants you will keep her from touching the "sterile" vaginal area. With each push, help direct her efforts. Keep her feet and legs relaxed. Between contractions, remind her to lie back and relax her whole body. She may enjoy ice chips and a cool cloth on her forehead. By now, your partner is so tuned in to your directions that it may be up to you to translate the doctor's instructions. Use clear, simple wording. When the crowning takes place, firmly direct her to drop the pushing position, open her mouth, and begin blowing. It may help to blow with her. If she feels stretching sensations, remind her that they are normal and everything is okay. When the baby is being born, remind her to keep her eyes open so she can see the birth of his head. Help with the next push as she expels the baby's body. Enjoy watching your baby being born.

PLACENTAL EXPULSION

Mother

Your baby is born, and you are flooded with feelings of relief, creativity, and joy. However, your work is not completely done. Your birthing attendant is concerned with one more important step, the delivery of the placenta. The moment your baby is delivered, the placenta starts to detach itself from its site on the uterine wall. With the next contraction, the placenta is naturally expelled. The attendant examines it carefully, making sure that no pieces are left inside the uterus to cause later hemorrhaging. Your uterus, cervix, vagina, perineum, and vulva are checked and, if necessary, repairs are made. If an episiotomy was performed, it is also repaired at this time. This period usually lasts from one to twenty minutes.

CONTRACTIONS

Your contractions will temporarily stop when your baby is born. When they resume they are usually mild, rhythmical, and painless.

POSSIBLE PHYSICAL CHANGES

Immediately after the birth of your baby, your uterus assumes a round shape and rises into your abdomen. As the placenta moves into your vagina you can see the umbilical cord lengthening. Following another mild contraction you can feel your placenta emerge painlessly from your vagina. You may experience a small trickle or a gush of blood. If you had an episiotomy, you may feel some sensation as it is being repaired. Some women have chills and trembling immediately after the birth of their child. You may be very thirsty and hungry, and want a nutritious snack.

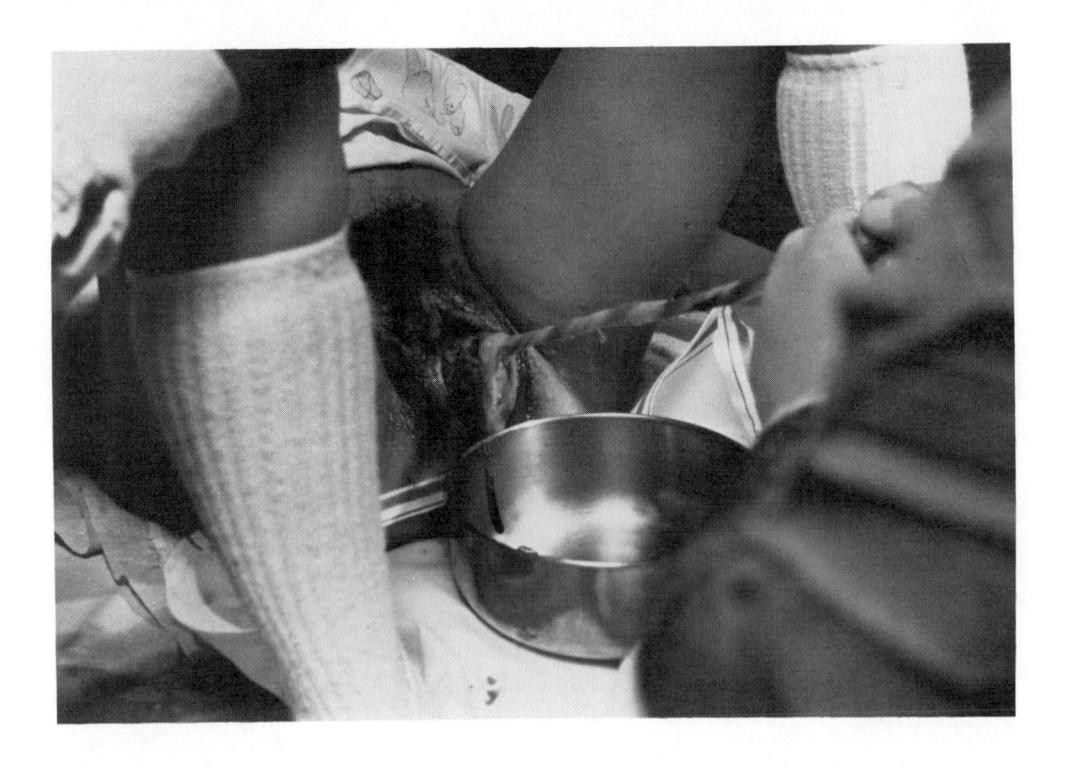

POSSIBLE EMOTIONAL CHANGES

There is no one right feeling after the birth of your baby. Depending on the length and difficulty of your labor, you may experience feelings ranging from ecstasy, joy, pride, happiness, delight, excitement, relief, surprise, and satisfaction to fatigue, anxiety, depression, or even disappointment. You may even experience all of these feelings at the same time.

WHAT TO DO

Although you may be more concerned with your baby at this time than with thinking about the placenta, you may be asked to give another little push to help deliver the placenta. When the placenta is delivered you may want to see this extraordinary organ, which has nourished your baby for nine months. If you have any questions, be sure to ask your attendants what they are doing to your body and why they are doing it.

Breathing. During the contractions of this stage, use your slow deep breathing. If you are shivering or trembling, take in a breath and let it out slowly between pursed lips. When you are asked to push, take in a deep breath and push down with your abdominal muscles.

Relaxation. Concentrate on relaxing your whole body after the birth of your baby. If you are shivering, concentrate on relaxing your thighs and legs. Remember to relax your pelvic floor as you are pushing the placenta out.

Position. If you are on a delivery table with your legs in stirrups, your legs may be very fatigued and you may experience cramps. Be sure to tell your birthing attendant and have him or her adjust the table.

Coach

She will need your instructions, encouragement, and support as she did during labor. Remind her that the last steps take only a few minutes and help her meet these last efforts with breathing and relaxation techniques. Understand that before she can begin to mother the baby she must first take care of her body and be assured that she has indeed survived physically and mentally. Give her a few minutes to regain her equilibrium. Tell her you love her.

COMFORTING TECHNIQUES

She may want ice chips or water to slake her thirst. A cool washcloth on her forehead may be refreshing. If she is shivering or trembling, stroking her legs or applying firm pressure on each side of her thighs may give her comfort. If she feels nauseated, suggest she take in a breath of air and let it out through pursed lips. If she needs to throw up, give her the basin and let her know it's okay and that the feeling will soon pass.

IMMEDIATE POSTPARTUM

Mother

Immediate postpartum, or the first hour after birth, is an important period both physically and emotionally. Physically, your body has worked very hard and is now making its first efforts to return to its nonpregnant state. Your blood pressure, pulse, and temperature will be monitored about every ten to fifteen minutes by your birthing attendant. These indicate how well your body systems are recovering. Blood and tissue will be expelled from the uterus and you will experience a heavy vaginal discharge. Your nurse or attendant will monitor it to be sure that the flow, color, and smell from the placental site are normal. Your bladder will be checked for fullness. Your uterus, cervix, vagina, perineum, and episiotomy site (if you had one) will be checked.

CONTRACTIONS

The most important thing that will happen naturally is the contraction of your uterine muscles to clamp down on the site where the placenta detached and prevent hemorrhaging. To keep the uterus firmly contracted, your nurse or birthing attendant will massage the uterus by hand; this may be painful. They will continue to check the fundus, or top of your uterus, to be sure that it is contracting and remaining firm. You will be given a sanitary pad for the vaginal flow and will be checked to see that there is no excessive bleeding or large blood clots. Some women, especially those who have had other births, may experience "afterpains" at this time. As the uterus contracts, the mother may experience quite painful sensations. When a mother breast-feeds, she may feel the contractions even more intensely.

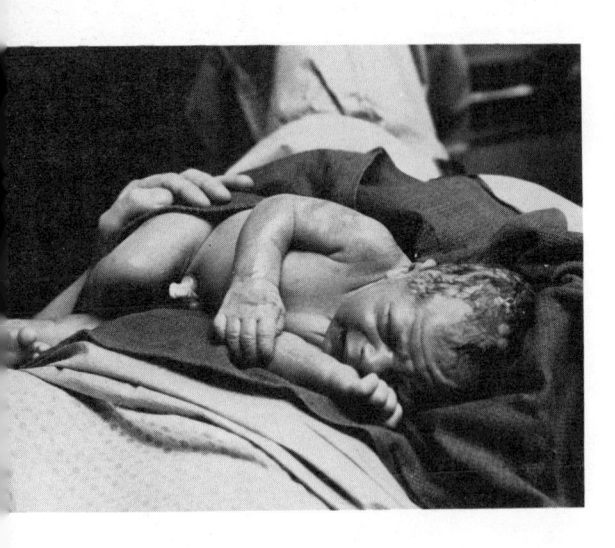

POSSIBLE PHYSICAL CHANGES

After the birth of your baby you will have contractions of varying intensity. You will also experience varying degrees of other pain and stress. If you had a long labor with a long delivery and large baby, you may be experiencing pain in your pelvis and vagina. If you had an episiotomy, you may feel pain or burning after the anesthetic wears off. It is not unusual to experience chills and trembling, and a warm blanket feels especially good. You will probably be very thirsty and may even have a ravenous appetite.

POSSIBLE EMOTIONAL CHANGES

You have survived an extraordinary experience. You now have time and energy to become acquainted with this new person you have conceived and given birth to. Depending on the length and difficulty of labor, all of the range of feelings you experienced at the birth of your child, from ecstasy to disappointment, may still be there.

When you are assured that your baby is okay, you will be eager to see, hold, feel, touch, and hear your baby. You may be overcome with a loving feeling for him, or you may need some time to become acquainted with this new person in your life. You may feel new and strong feelings of love and appreciation for your husband/coach who has stood by you and shared the birth of your baby.

WHAT TO DO

This is a special and private time for you and your baby. It is a privilege to get to know him. He is yours—forever. Do not be afraid of this hardy character who has been nine months in your body. Look at his hands, feet, and his body. Look into his eyes; you are the first person he has ever looked at. He will be fascinated with your eyes, your mouth, and your face. Talk to him; he will be fascinated with the first words he hears; he will love the sound and rhythm of your voice. Hold him, rock him, sing to him. These are the first and most important experiences of his life. Give him to his father and let his father get to know him as well.

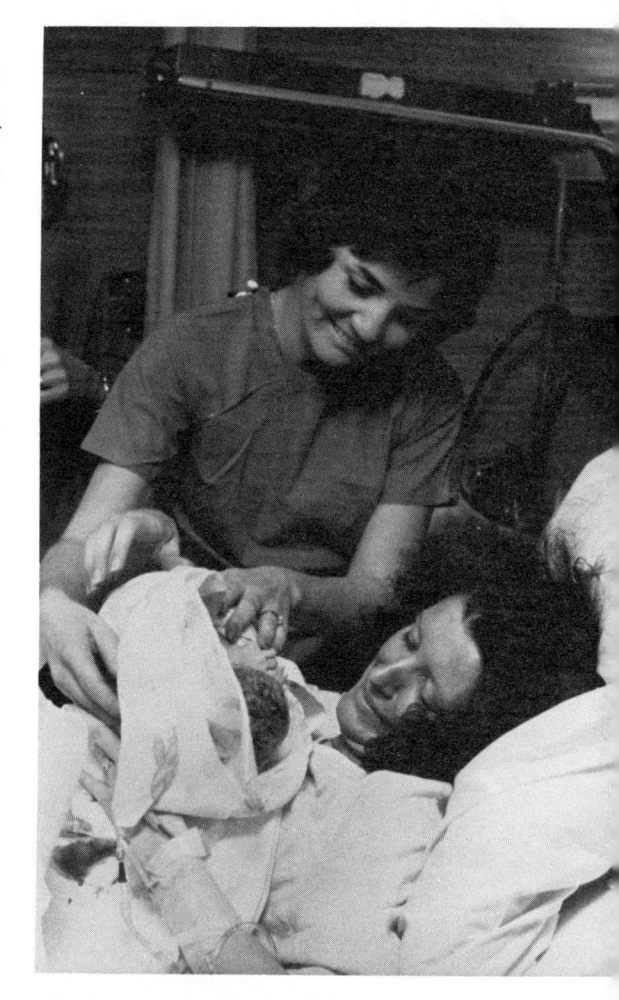

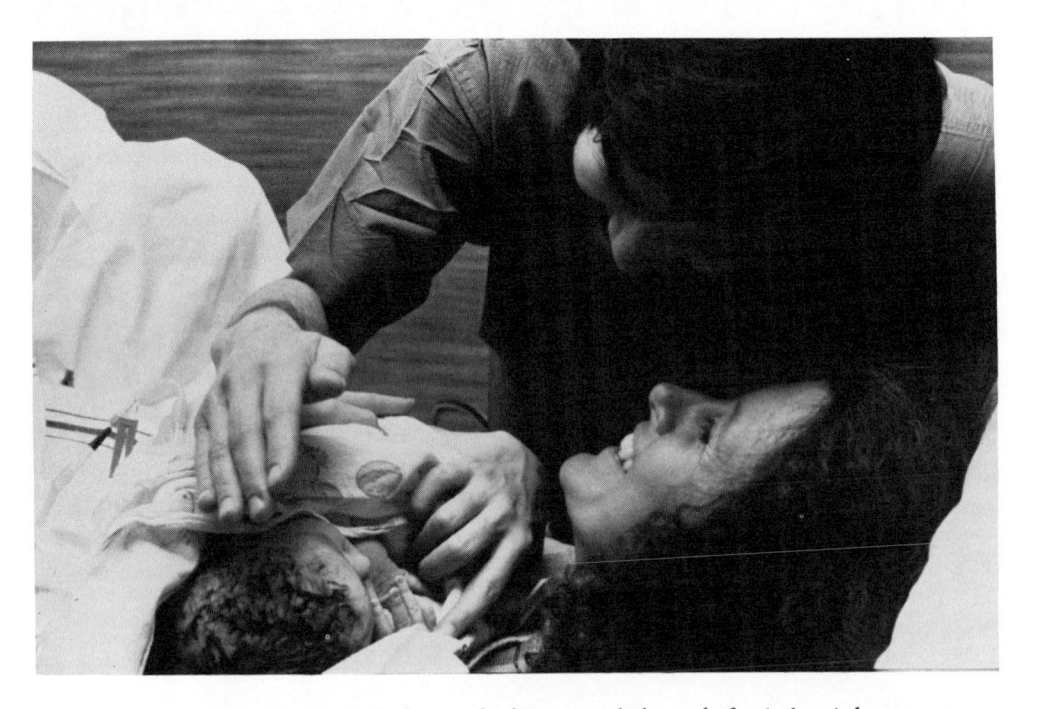

With your first experience in breast-feeding your baby, ask for help. Ask your attendant to get your baby in the right position to grasp your nipple. Ask him or her to help you in brushing your baby's cheek with your nipple and guiding it into his mouth. Do not be disappointed if your baby does not breast-feed right away. This is an exploratory time in which he is becoming accustomed to your feel, your taste, and your smell. Your baby will probably begin to lick at the nipple. This sets into action a whole physiological process that will signal your hormones to make your uterus contract, thus speeding your recovery.

Breathing. If you are experiencing painful contractions, use your slow deep breathing to match their intensity. Should they be quite painful, you may even want to use your accelerated breathing. If you experience chills or trembling, take in a deep breath, hold it, and then let it slowly escape from your lips.

Relaxation. If your contractions are painful, concentrate on relaxing your whole pelvic region. Stroking and massage may give you some relief. If the contractions get too painful, ask for medication.

Other. Be sure to drink plenty of fluids and try to empty your bladder as soon as possible. Once you are assured of both yours and your baby's health, you may experience an overwhelming desire to sleep. You have done a good job; you know your baby is okay and you now deserve a long rest.

Coach

Intense, mixed, and fluctuating feelings are all a part of the postpartum period. It is common for the coach/father to experience a range of feelings, from elation and ecstasy to depression. Depending on the length and difficulty of the labor, it will take some time to recover and reassure yourself that not only the mother but you have survived the experience intact. It is your task to allow the mother and yourself to experience your own feelings and accept your reactions for the moment, and to allow yourselves to change.

HOW TO HELP

During this time you have the task of helping the mother and yourself recover from labor, and experiencing the joy of receiving and exploring the new life that you have brought forth. Ask the birthing attendant to tell you what is going on with the mother's body and why certain procedures are being performed. Have the attendant answer your questions about the birth and your baby.

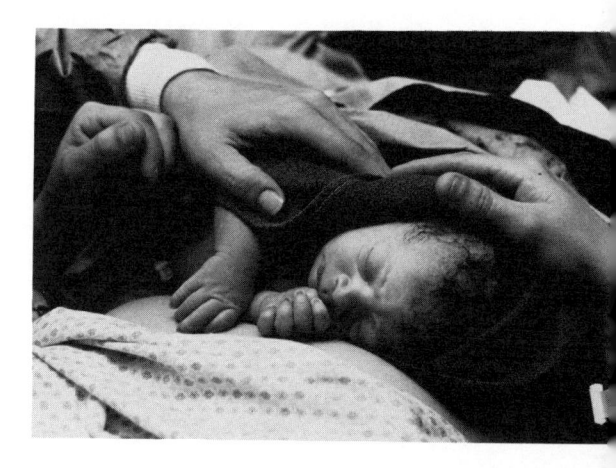

It is normal at this time for you both to relive the birth: what you both did, how it was helpful, what you might do for another labor. You will both appreciate the love, appreciation, and admiration that comes from experiencing labor and birth together. You will find yourself not only bonding to the new baby, but bonding to each other in a new and strengthened way. The new mother will be especially appreciative if you give her a few breathing moments to adjust to her new body and the rigors which she has just undergone before she takes on the role of mothering her baby.

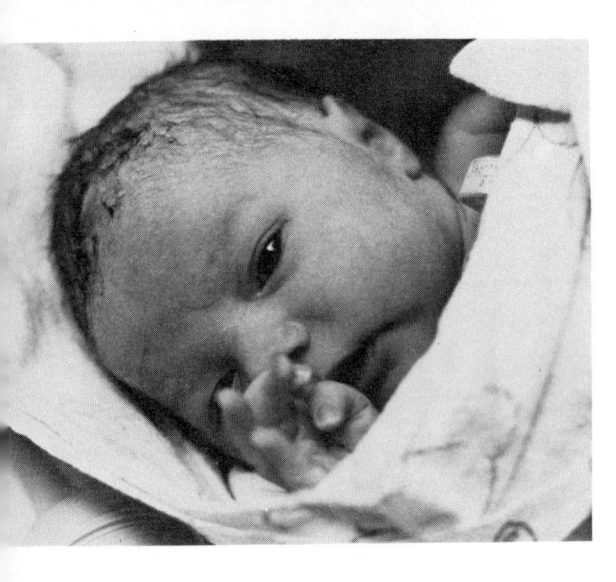

COMFORTING TECHNIQUES

Immediately following birth, a warm blanket may be very comforting for the mother. Ask for food and drink to refresh and revitalize her. Reassure her that both she and the baby are okay. If the mother wishes, wash her face and comb her hair.

After these moments, we do know that immediate contact between mother, father, and baby is very important in the development of your feelings for one another. This is the time for you to enjoy your new baby. It may be your task to make sure that the baby is given to the mother and that mother and baby can be together to get to know one another. Skin-to-skin contact helps ensure bonding and retention of the baby's body warmth. If the mother wishes to breast-feed, it may be your task to ask the nurse to help her. Breast-feeding is a learned task and, if she is a first-time breast-feeder, she will benefit from the physical and emotional help of the nursing staff.

The mother may be taken to the recovery room for observation for one or two hours. Be sure this includes you and the baby. Take this time to be alone with the mother and baby. He is your baby: explore his hands, fingers, body. Your baby can see and hear you. Look into his eyes, talk to him. Watch him look at you and listen to you. These are special moments that can never be repeated.

EARLY LABOR

WHAT IS HAPPENING
Effacement: 0–100%
Dilatation: 0–3 cm.
Duration: First labor 6–8 hrs.
　　　　　Subsequent labors 2–5 hrs.

CONTRACTIONS
Intensity: Mild
Length: 30–60 sec.
Intervals: 20–5 min. apart

POSSIBLE PHYSICAL SIGNS
Flulike feelings
Increased vaginal discharge
Menstrual-like cramps
Diarrhea
Low backache
Need to urinate
Increased pelvic pressure
Constipation

POSSIBLE EMOTIONAL CHANGES
"Nesting urge"
Excitement and anticipation
Apprehensive and anxious
Social
Relieved
Confident

MOTHER'S ROLE
Assess phase of labor
Maintain regular activities
Walk
Take warm shower
Talk
Rest as much as posible
Sleep if possible
Eat light energy food
Urinate every hour
Don't go to the hospital too early

BREATHING
Don't begin until you absolutely need to
Begin with slow deep breathing
Concentrate on focal point

RELAXATION
Begin active relaxation when needed
Concentrate on releasing tension

POSITION
Change position often; move and walk about

COACH'S ROLE
Help assess contractions
Help mother conserve energy
Offer moral support
Help find comfortable position
Conserve your own energy

ACTIVE LABOR

WHAT IS HAPPENING
Effacement: 100%
Dilatation: 3–7 cm.
Duration: First labor 3–6 hrs.
    Subsequent labors: 1–3 hrs.

CONTRACTIONS
Intensity: Increasingly stronger
Length: 45–60 sec.
Intervals: 5–3 min. apart

POSSIBLE PHYSICAL SIGNS
Gradual increase in bloody show
Discomfort in back, hips, legs
Cramping in feet or thighs
Need greater concentration to remain in control

POSSIBLE EMOTIONAL CHANGES
Become more serious, quiet
Preoccupied with work
Less sociable
Resent distractions
Doubt ability to cope with labor
Panic about being alone

MOTHER'S ROLE
Catch each contraction beginning
Match the intensity of each contraction
Concentrate on resting between contractions
Listen to your coach
Change position every half hour
Empty your bladder every hour

BREATHING
Switch to second phase breathing when needed
Concentrate on focal point
Use cleansing breath as signal to coach
Avoid hyperventilation

RELAXATION
Concentrate on relaxing with each inhalation
Tell your coach where you want massage and pressure

POSITION
Change every 30 minutes
Try side-lying, semi-sitting, all-fours, kneeling

COACH'S ROLE
Analyze effectiveness of your coaching techniques
If contractions are regular, time them
Keep mother informed about progress of labor
Reassure mother
Adjust pillows to give support
Massage sacrum, coccyx, hipbones, pubic bone when needed
Change massage techniques as labor progresses and baby moves down
Offer ice chips
Offer lollipops or tea with sugar
Suggest she use Chapstick or brush teeth
Keep up your energy with snacks
Empty your bladder when needed

TRANSITION

WHAT IS HAPPENING
Effacement: Complete
Dilatation: 7–10 cm.
Duration: First labor 10 min.–2 hrs.
  Subsequent labors: Same

CONTRACTIONS
Intensity: Extremely strong, erratic
Length: 60–90 sec.
Intervals: 3–1 min. (may piggyback)

POSSIBLE PHYSICAL SIGNS
Overwhelming desire to push
Pressure on pelvic floor
Pressure in rectum
Dark heavy mucous discharge
Hot flashes/cold chills
Cold feet
Desire to sleep and escape
Burping, hiccoughs, nausea, vomiting

POSSIBLE EMOTIONAL CHANGES
Loss of control
Restlessness and irritability
Panicky, discouraged
Fatigued and confused
Trapped and panicked
Need support
Turn inward

MOTHER'S ROLE
Remember, this is the shortest stage
Don't give up, you are not alone
Don't panic
Tension prolongs labor

BREATHING
Transitional breathing
Return to slow chest breathing when this no longer works
When desire to push becomes overwhelming, give several blows at peak of contractions
Concentrate on focal point
Listen to coach's directions

RELAXATION
Concentrate on coach's directions
Concentrate on coach's touch
Remember, tension will prolong labor
Relax pelvic floor and thighs
Relax face and shoulders

POSITION
Find position most comfortable
Try side-lying position, or all-fours

COACH'S ROLE
Don't panic—assure mother
Change into delivery room garb
Give encouragement, praise, support
Instruct her breathing and relaxation
Use eye contact
Use a firm voice
Take one contraction at a time
Try to remain calm and understanding
Use all massage techniques
Ask mother what gives her greatest comfort
Massage sacrum, coccyx, hipbone, pubic bone, and pelvic floor when needed
Stroke her face, neck, and shoulders between contractions
Try heat or cold in areas of discomfort
Put cold washcloth on forehead
Have her put on warm socks

DELIVERY

WHAT IS HAPPENING
Effacement: Complete
Dilatation: Complete
Duration: First baby: 1-2 hrs.
    Subsequeent babies: 15 min.-2 hrs.

CONTRACTIONS
Intensity: Less intense
Length: 60-90 sec.
Intervals: 1-3 min.

POSSIBLE PHYSICAL SIGNS
Rectal and perineal pressure
Perineal bulging
Shaking legs
Profuse bloody show
Active participation

POSSIBLE EMOTIONAL CHANGES
Increased alertness
Energy begins to return
Usually feels good to push
Excitement and exhilaration
Joy, awe, surprise, and fear

MOTHER'S ROLE
Do not push until cervix is completely dilated
Ask to see delivery
Get in a comfortable position
Concentrate on pushing baby down and out

BREATHING
Expulsion breathing
Concentrate
Hold breath as long as possible
When head crowns: lie back and begin panting

RELAXATION
Concentrate on relaxing pelvic floor, perineum, thighs and feet
Relax face and neck muscles when pushing

POSITION
Choose comfortable position: semi-sitting or side-lying
Tilt pelvic, relax perineum, back straight, shoulders rounded, arms out, neck and head erect

COACH'S ROLE
Be sure mother is in comfortable position
Stay with her as she is moved from labor to delivery room
Bring pillows with you
Ice chips will refresh her
Ask birthing attendant to be sure her legs are in a comfortable position
Remind her to relax between contractions
Help her stop pushing at the crowning
Enjoy the experience

PLACENTAL EXPULSION

WHAT IS HAPPENING
The placenta is detaching itself from the site in the uterus
The placenta is expelled through the vagina
Duration: 1–20 min.

CONTRACTIONS
Intensity: Mild
Length: Variable
Intervals: Variable

POSSIBLE PHYSICAL SIGNS
Uterus rises in abdomen
Umbilical cord lengthens
Placenta emerges
Mother becomes thirsty and hungry

POSSIBLE EMOTIONAL CHANGES
Wide range of feelings: ecstasy, joy, pride, happiness, delight, fatigue, anxiety, astonishment, etc.

MOTHER'S ROLE
Push to deliver placenta
Ask attendants what they are doing and why they are doing it

BREATHING
Slow deep breathing

RELAXATION
Concentrate on relaxing perineum and pelvic floor

POSITION
Be sure to ask your attendant to get you into a comfortable position

COACH'S ROLE
Give mother special support
Assure mother that everything is okay and that she has survived the experience
Ask doctor or nurse to explain what they are doing
Help with breathing and relaxation
Tell her you love her
Give ice chips or water
Cool washcloth on forehead

IMMEDIATE POSTPARTUM

WHAT IS HAPPENING
Uterus contracting, diminishing
Blood and tissue expelled from uterus
Episiotomy repair (if necessary)
"Afterpains"

CONTRACTIONS
Strength: Vary from slight to very strong (especially with subsequent labors and breast-feeding mothers)
Length: Variable
Intervals: Variable

POSSIBLE PHYSICAL SIGNS
Varying degrees of pain in pelvis and vagina and episiotomy site
Chills and trembling
Thirst and hunger

POSSIBLE EMOTIONAL SIGNS
Range of feelings from ecstasy to disappointment
Loving feelings and appreciation toward coach
Eager to see, feel, touch and hear baby

MOTHER'S ROLE
Ask for help in breast-feeding
Explore your baby
Talk to your baby
Establish eye contact
Hold, rock, and sing to baby

BREATHING
Use slow deep breathing if you need it
Hold breath if you have chills or trembling

RELAXATION
Concentrate on relaxing pelvic floor
Go to sleep when you are ready

COACH'S ROLE
Have birthing attendants tell both of you what is going on and answer questions about the birth and your baby
Ask for food, drink, and warm blanket for mother
Call family and friends
Wash mother's face and comb her hair
Ask for skin-to-skin contact for mother and baby
Explore your baby
Be sure that you, the mother, and baby have this special time together

10.

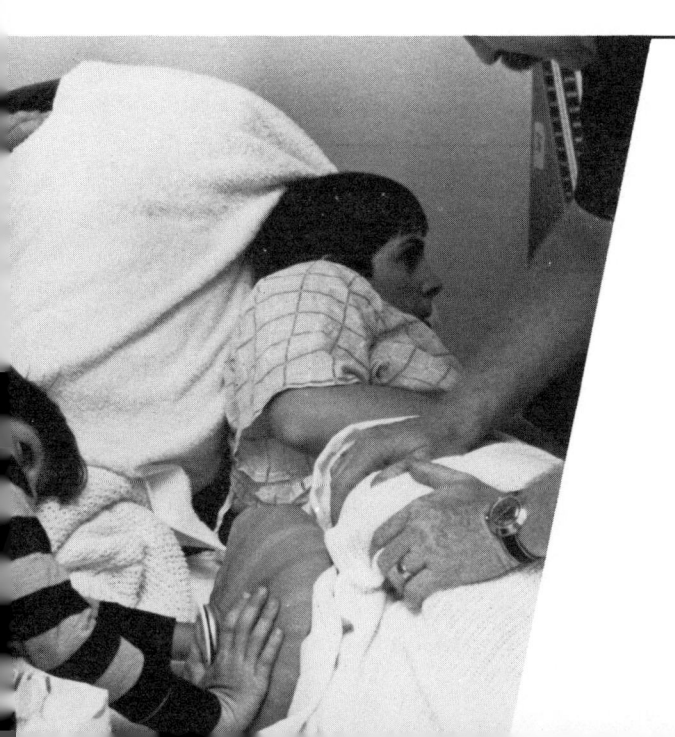

Family-centered Alternatives

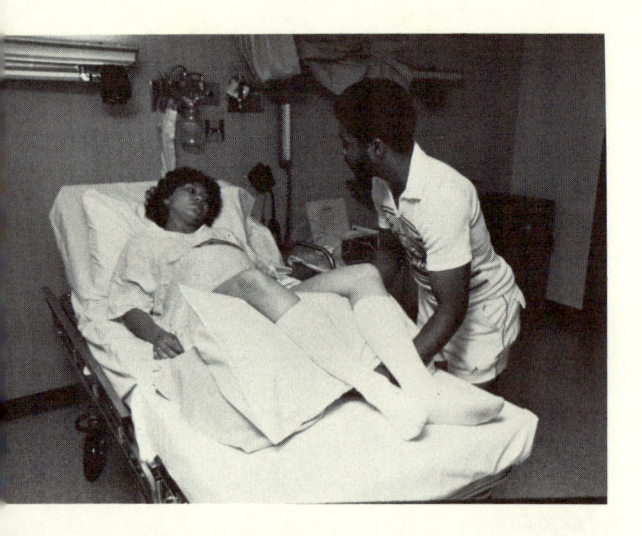

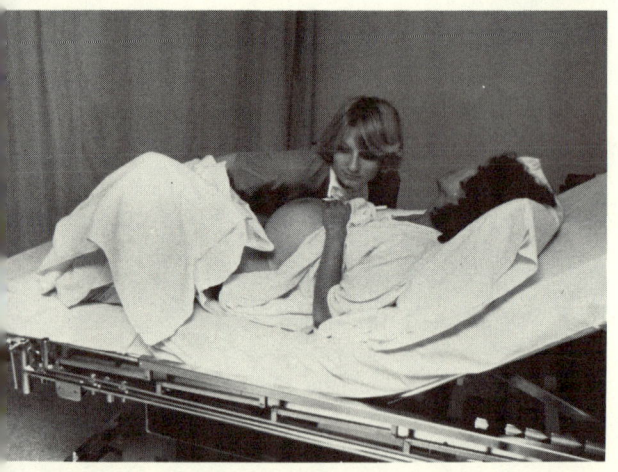

Family-centered maternity care is not an investment in wallpaper, beds, or floor plans, but a philosophy and attitude that looks at low-risk pregnancies and birth as natural biological functions that concern not only the birth of a baby, but the birth of a family. It can take place in a hospital, birthing room, birthing center, or at home.

BIRTHING ROOM

One of the most popular alternatives in many hospitals is the birthing room. Anita and Andre have chosen to have their child in a birthing room at a hospital where they can labor and deliver their baby and recover in the same place.

The birthing room provides a pleasant, comfortable atmosphere in which to give birth and eliminates the disruptive moves from labor to delivery to recovery room. It has the advantages of a comfortable environment combined with the back-up support of a medical facility.

Special efforts have been made to make the birthing room as comfortable as possible. Any instruments that might be needed for an emergency are easily accessible. This is the room where Anita and Andre will spend the next eight hours giving birth to their baby.

A supportive staff is an important element of the birthing-room concept. Anita and Andre are treated with respect and dignity. Andre has been trained to help Anita cope with the contractions of labor and birth.

Anita's doctor has not prescribed a prep, enema, or IV solution. Many institutions are now questioning the value of these routines, which most women receive automatically upon admission to the hospital.

Andre gives Anita a popsicle to moisten her mouth, refresh her, and give her energy for the next contraction. During labor and birth, Anita's comfort is a major priority. She is not treated as a patient, but as a person involved in one of the most important acts of her life. Pillows and supports are given as needed. Popsicles, ice, washcloths, heating pads, juice, and liquids are offered to refresh and comfort her.

Anita's doctor will not prescribe the routine use of pitocin to augment labor. In normal births, its use may cause an increase in both the frequency and the intensity of contractions, and may lead to a drop in the fetal heart rate.

113

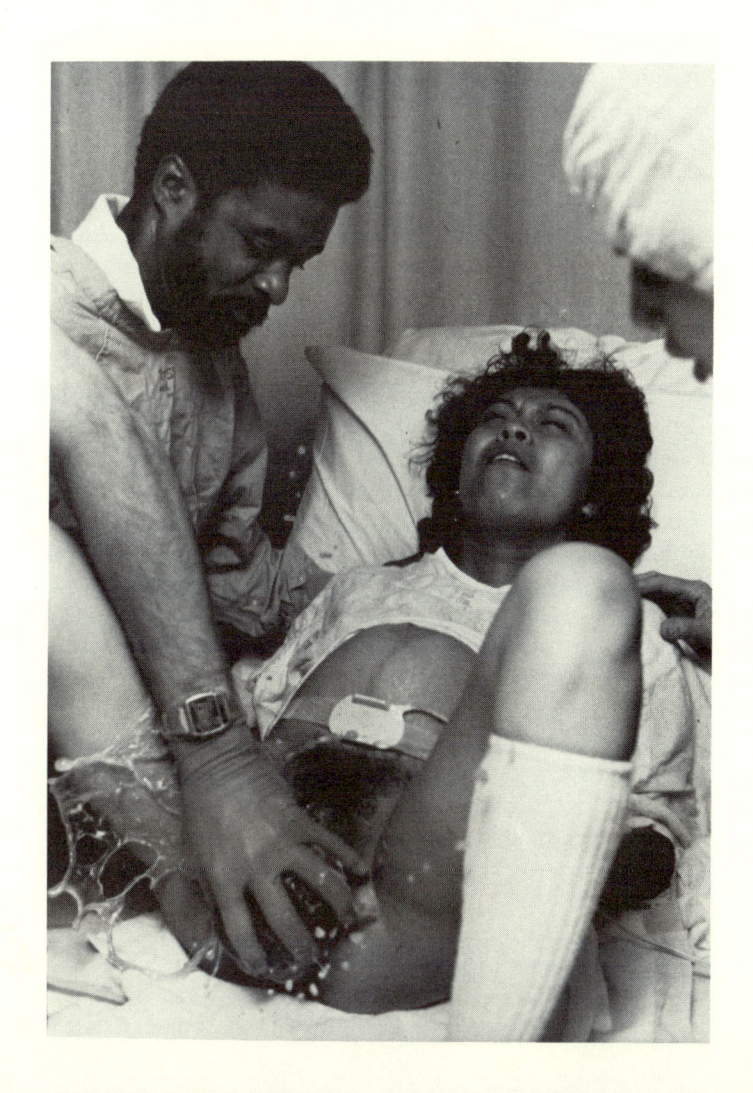

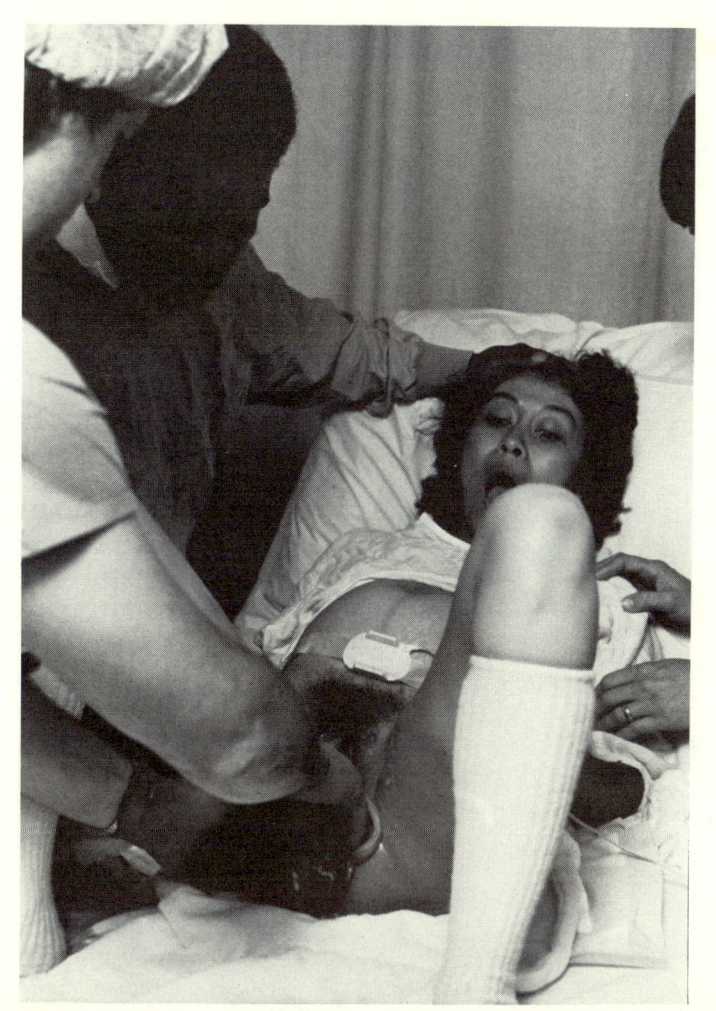

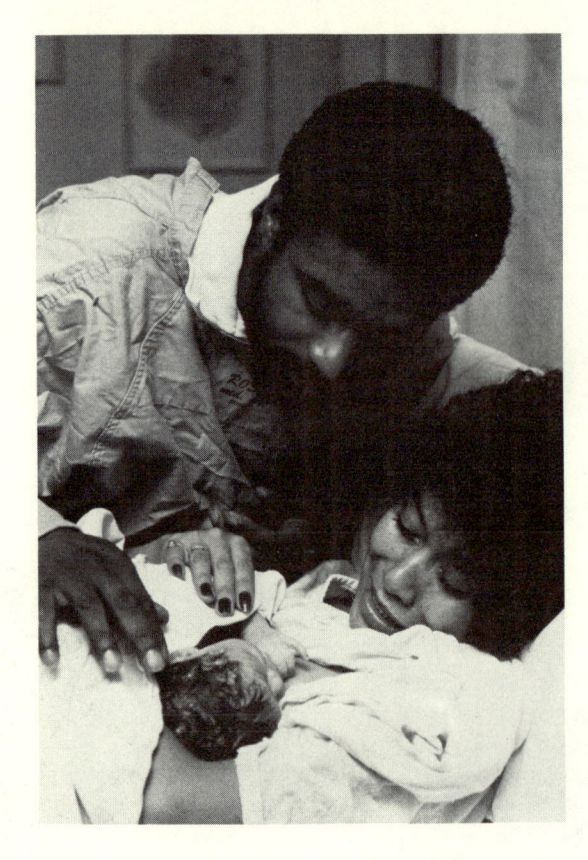

With family-centered maternity care, the use of anesthetics in a normal, uncomplicated birth is carefully evaluated. Any drug given in labor can affect the fetus and the woman's control. These drugs alter not only the mother's capacity for early interaction, but that of the newborn as well.

Anita is the one who can best choose the position most comfortable to her during labor and birth. Although some women find lying on the side more comfortable, Anita prefers to remain on her back in a semi-sitting position. When a woman is allowed to labor in a vertical position—either standing, sitting, or squatting—her contractions are more effective, her labor progresses faster, and she experiences less pain.

As she pushes, Anita's membranes rupture spontaneously. Although the early artificial rupture of membranes may shorten the duration of labor, it completely changes the normal physiology of labor. Intact membranes help protect the fetal head and prevent compression of the umbilical cord between the fetus and the uterus.

Anita has no need for a routine episiotomy, a small surgical cut made in the perineum that allows more room for the baby's delivery. In family-centered maternity care, episiotomies, unless they are indicated for fetal or maternal reasons, are avoided. They not only increase the blood loss of the mother, but make postpartum recovery less comfortable.

Anita is trained to open her mouth and pant when the largest part of her baby's head is at the opening. Immediately after birth, Alisha is handed to Anita, and skin-to-skin contact is encouraged. There is no separation from the baby for either mother or father. Privacy is given to the family so that they can share this time alone.

Since Anita chooses to breast-feed, her baby is put to her breast to nuzzle, root, and lick. Although Alisha might not breast-feed right away, this starts the process and that helps ensure successful breast-feeding. As Alisha licks the nipple, it causes a secretion of the hormone oxytocin into her mother's bloodstream, which causes the uterus to contract—facilitating placental separation and expulsion and thereby reducing postpartum bleeding.

The first minutes and hours of a baby's life are a sensitive period. When the baby, mother, and father share this early period together in privacy and close contact, there is an optimum opportunity for developing a special feeling of closeness. Because visual contact is so important, the routine procedure of putting silver nitrate in Alisha's eyes is delayed for the first hour, and can be delayed for four to six hours—perhaps more. There is no bathing to remove the vernix from the body.

BIRTHING CENTER (IN HOSPITAL)

The birthing center within the hospital is another alternative that offers a homelike birth facility allowing family and friends to be with the mother during labor and birth. Ann and K.L. have chosen to have their fourth baby in such a birthing center, where she will labor and deliver and stay with her baby in the same room.

Ann and K.L. have been Lamaze prenatal instructors for several years, and are prepared to be active participants in the birth of their fourth baby. The birthing center allows them to remain in control of their environment. They choose the support people whom they wish to have. The family is a unit and can have immediate and continuous contact with their baby.

Ann's primary care is provided by a certified nurse midwife, who has cared for Ann throughout her pregnancy. Ann may move about freely, eat, and drink, and do whatever is comfortable for her.

Ann's children will participate, and have been prepared ahead of time to know what to expect. Each child has an accompanying adult friend to attend to his or her own particular needs.

As knowledgable participants, Ann and K.L. are kept informed on the progress of their labor. If problems arise, specialized high-risk facilities and staff are only a few feet away. Ann's attending obstetrician is part of the hospital team available for consultation and assistance, should it be needed.

Ann is encouraged to keep active during the first phase of her labor. Walking about and a change of scenery help pass the time. Ann may be up and around for as long as she likes.

As her labor progresses, she is able to choose the position most comfortable for her, and there are few interventions in her normal labor pattern.

Hot tea and honey help to keep her refreshed and nourished. She finds it refreshing to

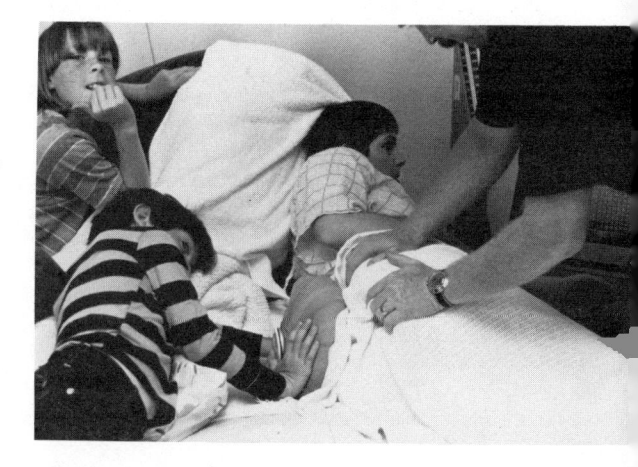

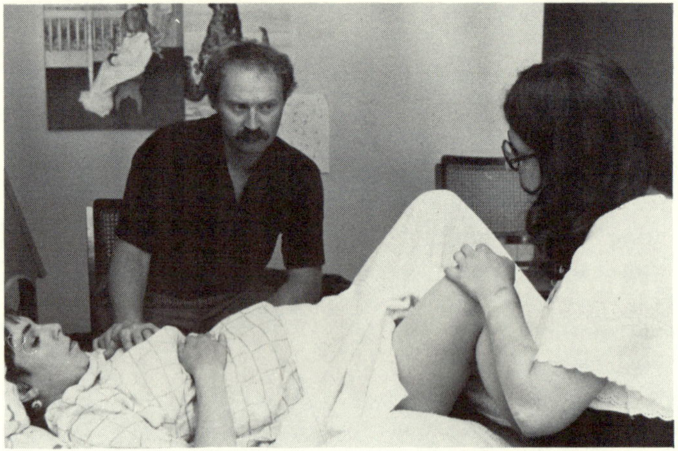

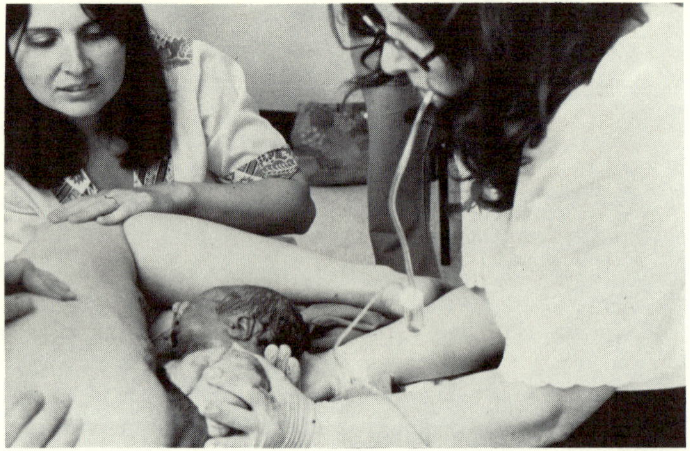

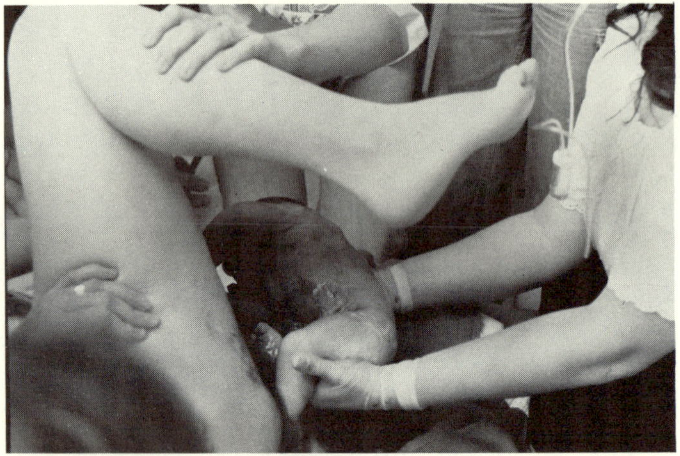

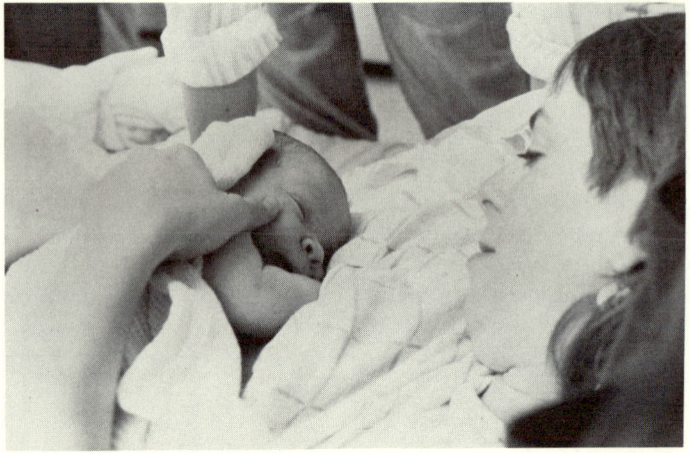

brush her teeth between contractions, and applies Chapstick to refresh her mouth and prevent her lips from drying out.

Ann and K.L. wait for the next contraction. Sitting in an upright position allows gravity to help Ann's baby move down; and, for the moment, gives her the greatest comfort.

As the baby moves down Ann feels greater pressure on her back and turns to her side for relief. Her son applies heat to her back while K.L. kneads her buttocks.

Experiencing back discomfort, Ann finds the knee/chest position against a bean bag support gives her some relief. All of the family pitches in to give her comfort. Her head is wiped with a cloth; her son, Jason, holds a heating pad on her tailbone as K.L. massages her thighs.

Jessica tries to comfort her mother during the most difficult stage of labor—transition. When Ann feels an urge to push, the nurse midwife checks her progress. She is completely dilated and ready to push.

As Ann delivers the head of the baby, she finds her pushing is more effective and comfortable in the side position.

With another push, the head emerges.

And moments later a son, Colin, is born.

K.L. cuts the cord and clamps it.

Colin is laid at Ann's breast, where he receives his first important skin-to-skin contact.

The family welcomes their new brother. After the birth, Ann stays in the center for less than twenty-four hours; she will have home visits from the nurse midwife afterward.

FREE-STANDING BIRTHING CENTERS

For couples who choose to deliver outside an institution, free-standing birthing centers are another alternative to the traditional hospital birth. The out-of-hospital birth center is staffed by certified nurse midwives. It offers total prenatal care, labor, and birth at the facility, and two home visits during the first four days after birth.

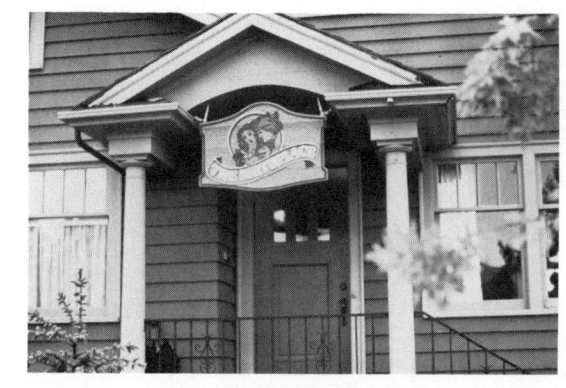

The homelike facilities are run by a team with physicians, midwives, and childbirth educators in consultation. Should an emergency arise, they are backed up by hospitals. Prevention of problems through education and health maintenance is emphasized. Classes in prenatal and postnatal care are given.

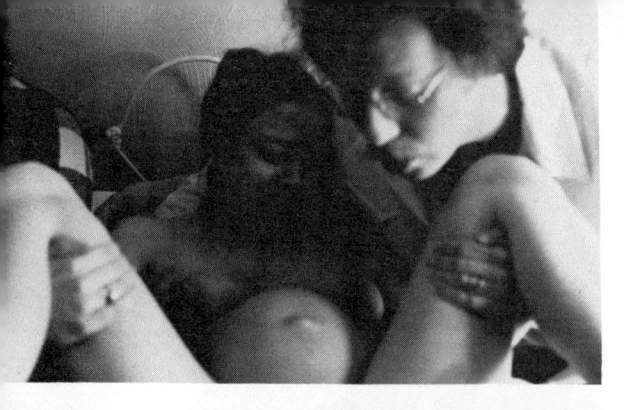

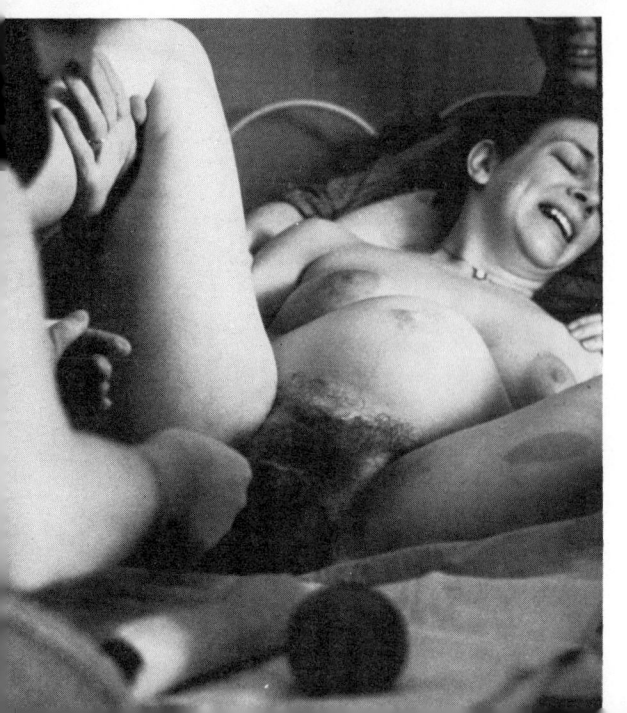

The purpose of the birthing center is to reinforce the confidence of couples in their ability to bear and raise healthy babies. It views couples as essential members of the health care team who share in decisions concerning their childbirth experience. Strict screening criteria are used to select mothers who are elegible to participate in the birth center. The women come from standard prenatal visits. Parents are encouraged to participate fully in their own health care.

The physical surroundings are homelike. The labor rooms are informal, with pictures, plants, reclining chairs, and dimmed lighting available. A warm, relaxed, family-centered atmosphere is the main focus.

Tucked away in a cupboard in each room is equipment needed for birth. In the white placenta basin there are cord clamps, sterile towels, scissors, and a bulb syringe for suctioning.

When Janet and Don arrive at The Birthplace, the midwife checks Janet's dilatation to ascertain that she is in active labor.

The midwife stays close by, interfering as little as possible. She watches Janet's progress closely, listens to the baby's heart tones and takes Janet's blood pressure every fifteen minutes, observes her behavioral responses, and checks her cervical dilatation to monitor for progress. Janet is given ice chips and fruit juices from the kitchen, and has cold washclothes for her head.

During their labor, Janet and Don work together during each contraction. Throughout the labor, she receives encouragement from her supporting team.

When Janet feels the urge to push, the midwife checks her and tells her that she is fully dilated and may push with the next contraction. Each push brings Janet's baby down. Don works with her through each contraction, and the midwife watches and guides the progress of the baby.

After trying several positions, Janet finds pushing more comfortable and effective in a side-lying position.

The midwife tells Janet that with the next contraction her baby's head will emerge and to stop pushing when she tells her to. When the next contraction comes, Janet pushes; as the baby's head emerges, she stops pushing and begins panting.

When the midwife asks Janet for a little push, the rest of her baby emerges. Don beams as he views his new baby daughter, Emily. The midwife takes a quick assessment of the baby.

Emily is handed to Janet and laid close to her body for skin-to-skin contact. Janet and Don look on as their baby snuggles on Janet's breast. The birth event itself, for most prepared parents, is a peak experience and is usually followed by a period of unreserved ecstasy. It is an emotional time, when feelings of relief and joy in the beauty of creation pervade the atmosphere.

HOME BIRTHS

A further alternative that some couples are exploring is the home birth with a physician or certified nurse midwife attending. It is important that home birth only be considered in areas of the country where medical support and back-up care ensure safety for the mother and baby.

Roberta and Bob have chosen to have their child at home. Roberta has experienced three normal, easy births in the hospital. So far, she's had a normal, healthy pregnancy. She anticipates this fourth birth will be a normal one.

Roberta is a healthy woman with an uncomplicated obstetrical history. She lives close to a major medical center and to an obstetrician and pediatrician who offer enthusiastic support. Roberta has been screened for any type of medical problem and has a history of no previous complications. In addition to Bob, she will be tended by a physician, an obstetrical nurse, several assistants, and her childbirth educator.

Her doctor is specially prepared with training and equipment to recognize and cope with any deviation from the normal. She is well aware of potential risks and has made careful provisions for medical backup. In the case of any fetal or maternal distress, she has made preparations to transfer Roberta to the nearby hospital for further evaluation.

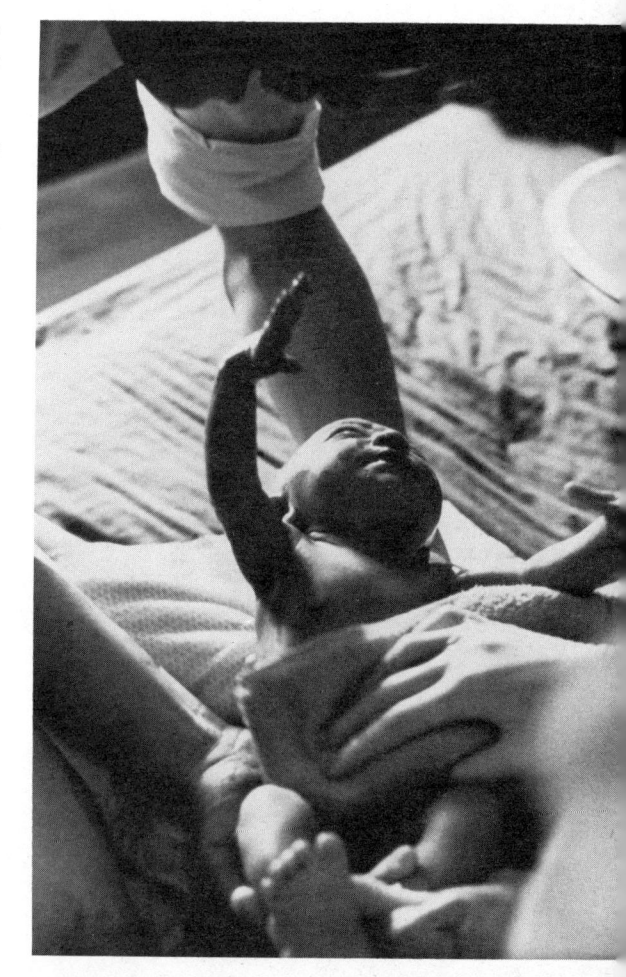

Bob is a medical doctor and both he and Roberta are knowledgeable about the life-threatening risks that may arise in labor and that cannot be predicted in advance. The most common risks are: fetal distress, a cord prolapse, and newborn asphyxia, which are life-threatening to the baby; and a postpartum hemorrhage, which is life-threatening to the mother. It is essential for Roberta and Bob to understand that if such complications arise without speedy access to emergency facilities the result may be a less than perfect outcome for the baby and/or the mother.

Roberta has put on a soft, comfortable nightgown. Her attendants help comfort her with pillows and loose covers. The labor will take place in a quiet, dimly lit room. They have prepared clean sheets, bedding, towels, and bowls. The doctor has brought her own scissors, aspirator, and other surgical supplies.

The children have been prepared for the birth, and each child has an adult to be with throughout the experience.

At the end of the first stage, Roberta begins to feel the contractions more acutely. She starts trembling and becomes nauseated during transition.

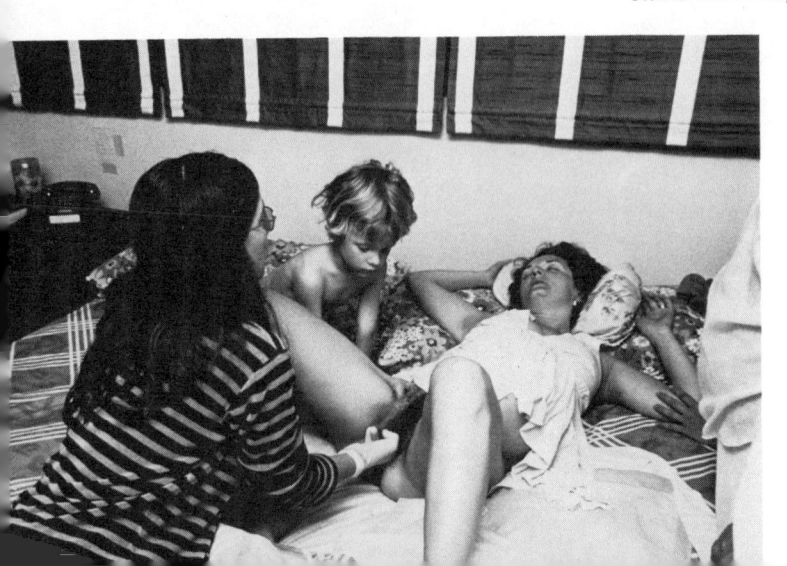

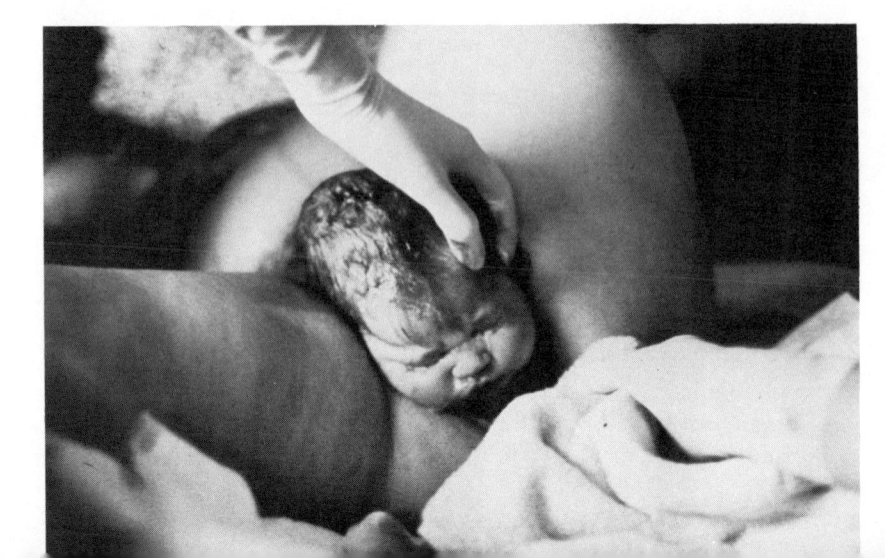

The doctor examines Roberta's progress and find that she is fully dilated and may now begin to push.

The birth attendants help Roberta into a side-lying position. As Roberta begins pushing, Bob helps guide the baby's head.

Roberta feels a burning, stretching sensation as the baby's head presses against her perineum. She stops pushing, leans back and relaxes as Bob delivers the head.

With the next push, Amanda is born and placed on her mother's breast. Her brothers are wide awake with joy and excitement.

At her mother's breast, Amanda licks her mother's nipple and begins to nurse. This is a special and unhurried time for Roberta and Amanda in which they are surrounded by people they love.

Roberta and Bob place Amanda in a bath that has been carefully warmed to the temperature of her body. She settles comfortably into the water and begins to coo.

Eyes wide, she stares at the outside world with great intensity, gathering her first impressions.

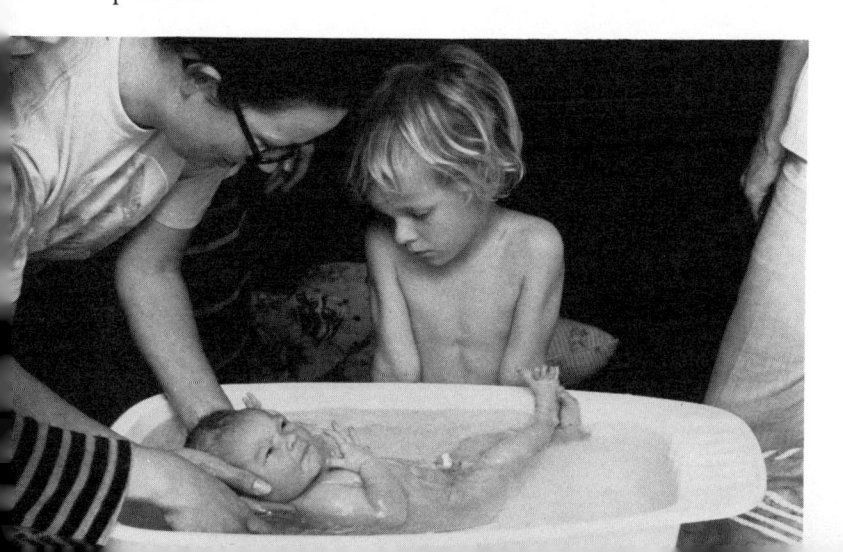

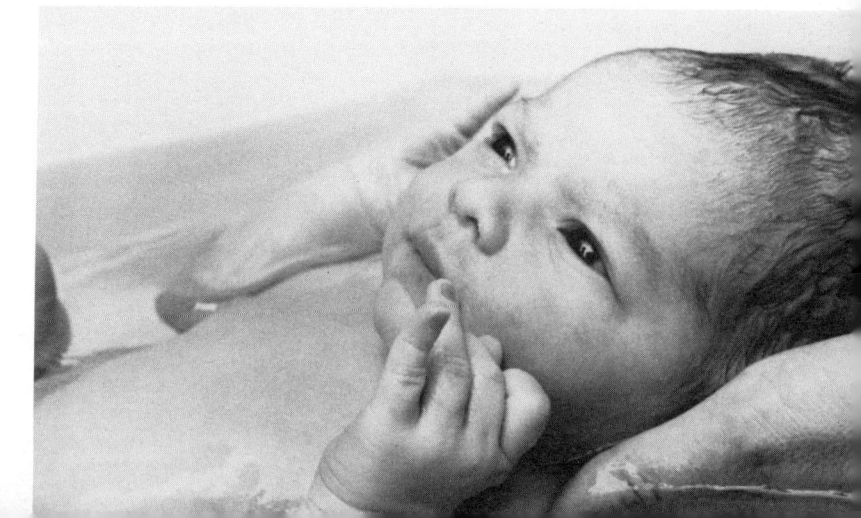

Her brother gazes back, and the two of them begin a relationship which will last a lifetime.

Amanda is wrapped in a warm blanket and admired by her father and sister.

She is then handed to her sister and brother, who gaze intently at their new sister and joyously welcome her into the family.

Grandmother, mother, and daughter celebrate the birth of Amanda. Once again, childbirth has become a family affair with its lore handed down from generation to generation, from mother to daughter.

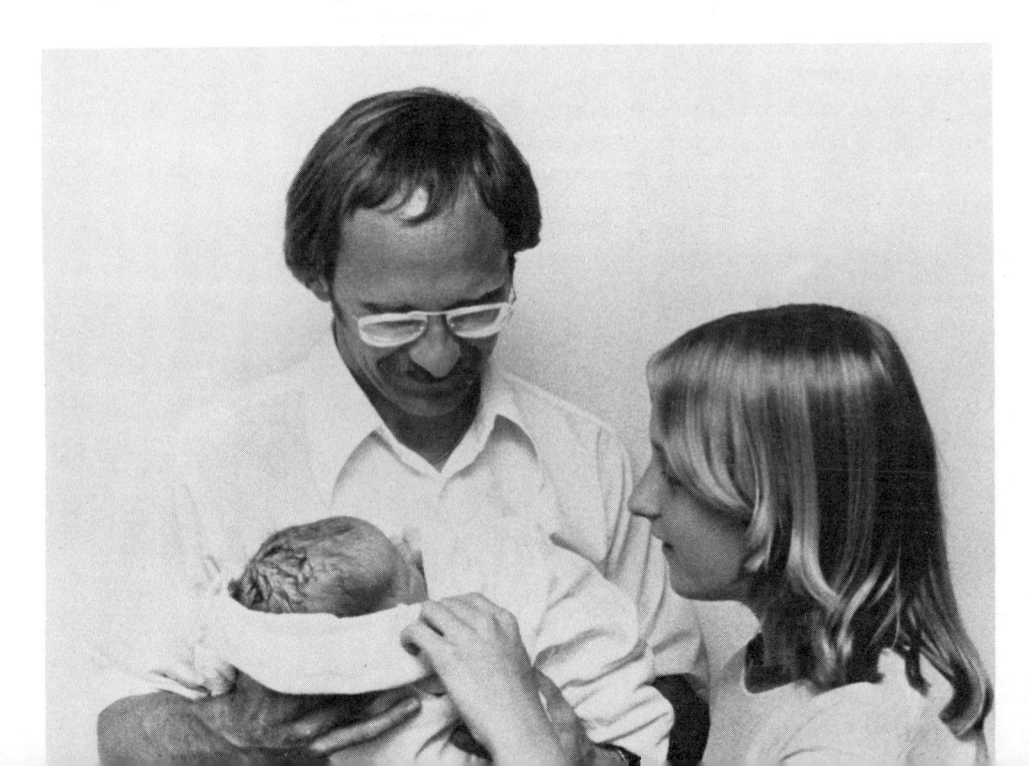

11.

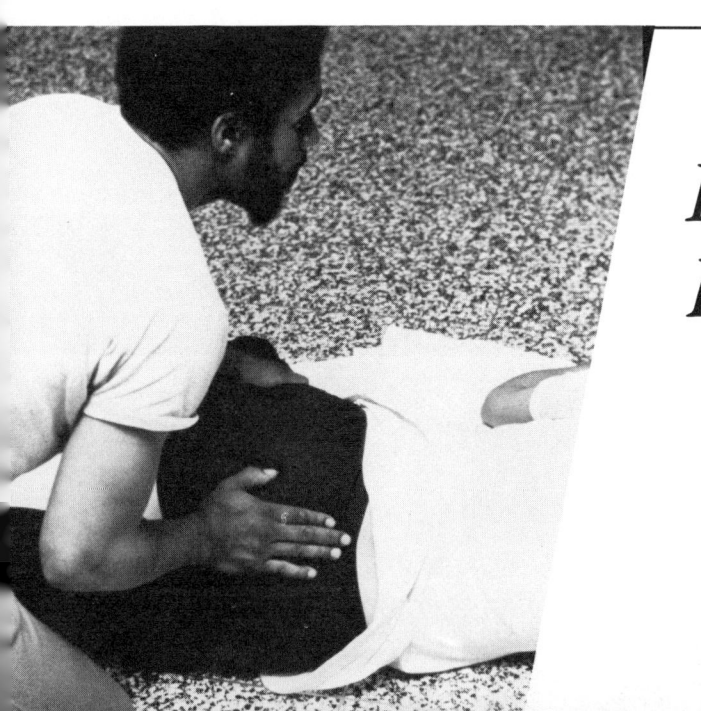

Possible Problems in Labor and Birth

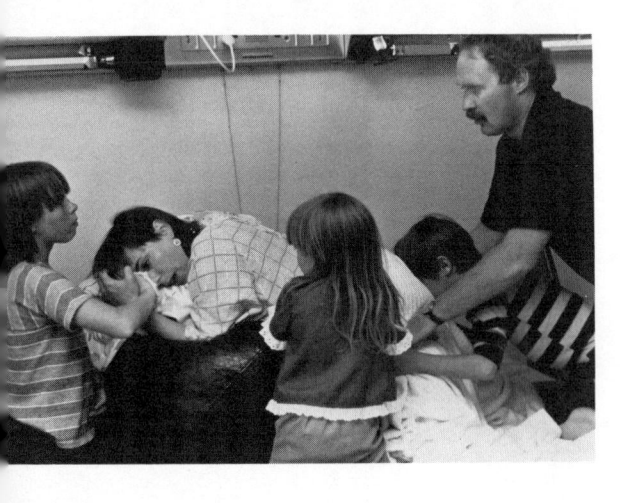

Although 95 percent of all labors are normal, being prepared means being aware of the kind of problems that may occur, along with the knowledge that you can take an active role in coping with them and the realization that at times only medical intervention can ensure the safety of you and your baby.

No two labors are exactly the same. Throughout labor and delivery a subtle relationship exists between the passenger, and passageway, and the powers of the contractions. Variations in labor and delivery patterns occur when there is a disproportion between the passageway and the passenger, or when the uterine contractions are ineffective, erratic, or excessive.

Passageway

A relative disproportion between the size and shape of your pelvis and the size of your baby may slow dilatation or stop it completely even though contractions continue. If this happens, medical intervention is necessary and a cesarean delivery is usually indicated.

Passenger

The size, position, and presentation of your baby may result in variations that call for medical intervention. If the baby is too large for your pelvis, cesarean section is indicated. If the baby is in a breech presentation or posterior position, labor may be prolonged and you may experience back discomfort. Forceps may be used to assist in the birth. Brow or shoulder presentations are indicators of a cesarean section; some hospitals section all breech presentations.

Powers

Uterine contractions not only thin and open the cervix but also help to expel the baby. If they are ineffective, weak, or infrequent (uterine inertia) or if the uterus fails to dilate effectively (distoria), you may require some kind of medication. Contractions may be erratic, originating in the lower part of the uterus instead of the top, resulting in ineffectual labor. If contractions are uncoordinated, they are difficult to predict and control.

BACK LABOR

If your baby is in a posterior or a breech position, you are more apt to experience back pain during labor. When the back of your baby's head is pressed against your sacrum, you will probably feel discomfort as the bony parts come together with each contraction. In late dilatation or transition, as the baby descends, back labor may occur no matter what the presentation. Just before crowning, you may experience backache as your baby presses against your sacrum and coccyx.

If you have more backaches in the last week of pregnancy, especially at night or early in the morning, it may be a sign that you are going to experience back labor. Irregular contractions during the second phase of active labor, contractions felt in the sacrum and buttocks, and occasional pains in the legs may be indications that the baby is in a posterior position.

Because the contractions are felt in the back, you may have more difficulty in relaxing and may be restless and irritable. If, as your baby comes down in the posterior position, he does not rotate to the anterior position, you will have a longer and more fatiguing pushing stage.

Your goal during back labor is to try to find a position that will give you relief and help your baby to rotate to the anterior position. Since lying flat on your back is probably the least effective position to accomplish this, alternate the upright, kneeling, side-lying and all-fours positions during your labor. Try sitting straight up with your legs crossed or tucked beneath you. Putting pillows in front of you, or using your bed table, lean forward to relieve pressure on your back. If this doesn't give you comfort, try putting pillows or a bean bag chair in front of you, get into a kneeling position and, again, lean forward as far as possible.

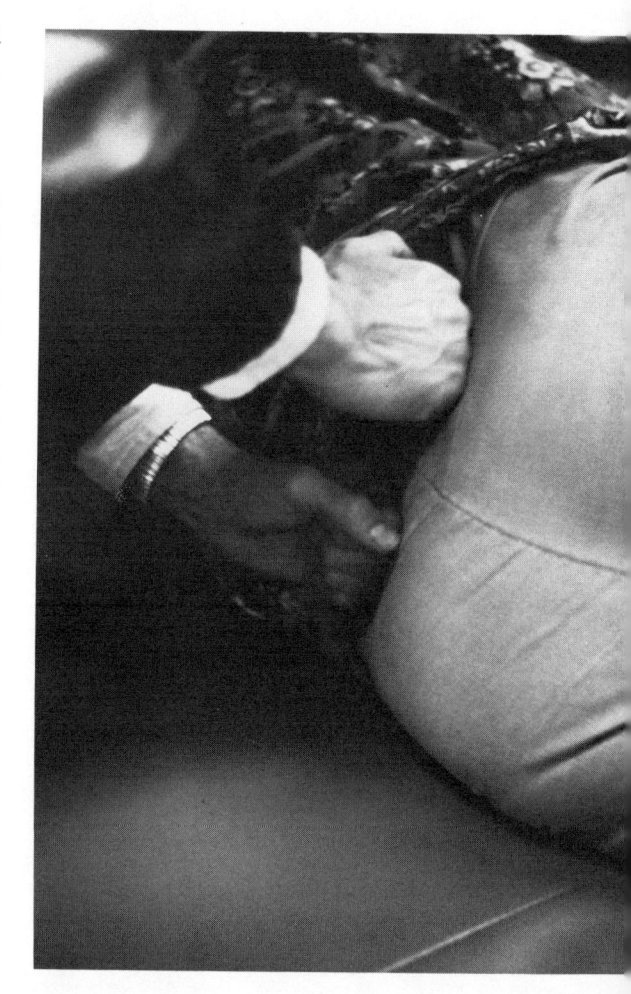

Try the side-lying position, lying on the side opposite your baby's back with your upper leg bent and leaning on the bed (if your baby's back is on your right side, lie on your left side). You may find that getting on all fours and rocking back and forth will give you some relief. Even standing and walking around (if your membranes have not ruptured) may be more comfortable and help to turn your baby. Be sure you change positions every half hour.

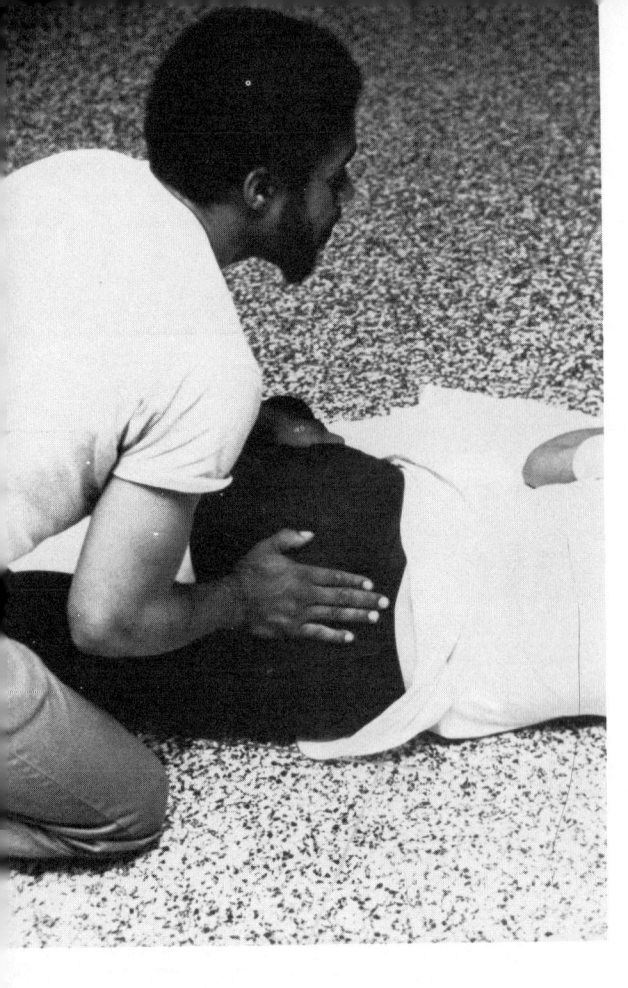

Coach

The coach should utilize all the massage techniques. Change them as the baby moves down. Try very firm pressure on both sides of the sacrum, the center of the sacrum, and deep down on the coccyx. Kneading the hip joints and buttocks may give relief. You may find that several persons massaging several different places will give the mother the greatest comfort.

A hot (not burning) washcloth, towel, or hot water bottle on all the pressure points may feel good. You can also try a cloth or towel soaked in cold water (or, place ice chips in the folds) or even a cold pack. Remember to keep a cool cloth on her head if she is hot.

Coaching is especially important with back labor. Although breathing and relaxation techniques will be harder for the woman with back labor, they are twice as important. Make her concentrate on her techniques to distract her attention from her discomfort. Relaxation of the pelvic joints is especially important.

The woman with back labor cannot be left alone. She needs as much physical, verbal, and emotional help as she can get from as many people as can give it. She needs to know why she is experiencing discomfort and be given special support and encouragement for the extra effort that it takes on her part.

12.

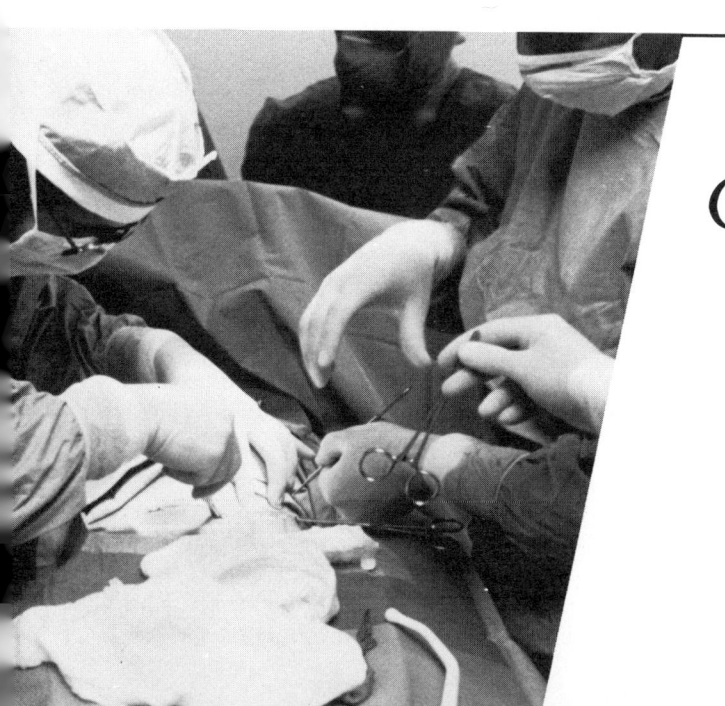

Cesarean Childbirth

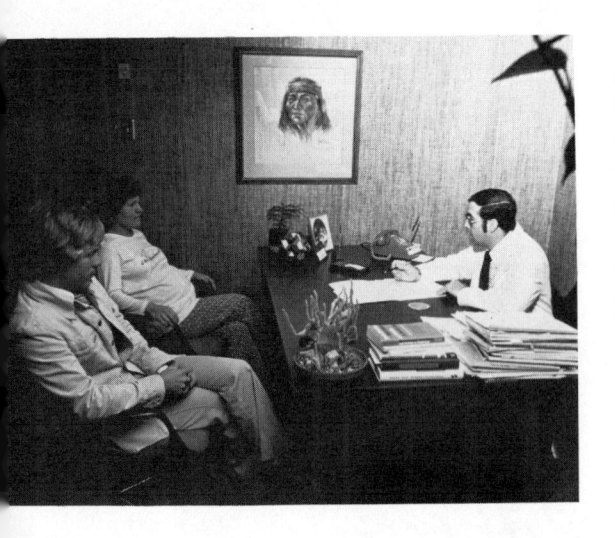

You have the hopes and concerns of all new parents. Your first priority is a healthy and safe birth experience for you and your baby. Although every woman expects a normal, uncomplicated pregnancy, you have at least one chance in ten of having a cesarean delivery. For the unprepared mother, a cesarean can be a frightening, disappointing, and depressing experience. With preparation, cesarean birth can be a shared, family-centered experience in which both the father and the mother can welcome the baby into the world.

Forty years ago cesarean births were rare. Today they are on the increase. This seems to be the result of advances in surgical technique, anesthesia, and antibiotics. For the surgeon, a cesarean operation is usually a routine procedure. For the mother, father, and baby, a cesarean childbirth has significance beyond the birth itself.

Cesarean childbirth was known long before the Romans. Contrary to popular belief, the word "cesarean" does not come from Julius Caesar. It is derived from the Latin word "caedere" which means "to cut." A cesarean delivery was originally used only for a baby whose mother did not survive childbirth. The Roman statesman, Pompey, decreed that if a mother died in childbirth, the child should be surgically removed from the mother's abdomen to permit separate burial. The first successful live cesarean section took place in the 1500s when a farmer surgically removed the baby from his wife's body after midwives and surgeons had given her up for lost. The mother lived to the age of 77.

Today, parents want to be active participants in the birth of their baby and have choices and control over the birth. Parents who deliver by cesarean have some choice in the timing of the birth, the kind of anesthesia used, and whether or not the father will be present. Active participation by you, the parents, helps to establish family bonding among mother, father, and baby which, with cesarean childbirth, is as important as in vaginal childbirth.

As you prepare for your cesarean delivery you may wish to explore family-centered maternity care. Depending on the reason for your cesarean, you, the mother, may choose to remain awake during the entire procedure so you can be together with the father for the birth of your baby. Your arms are not strapped down, and you are able to see, hold, and nurse your baby if you wish. The baby's father may be with you during recovery. You may be able to room in, breast-feed, and have your other children visit you. However, you should know that, should an emergency situation arise, the safety and health of you and your baby will take precedence over any options you may have discussed with your doctor.

When you go for your prenatal examination, be sure your baby's father goes too. This is a significant step toward family-centered health care. Part of the father's role is to understand and support you during your pregnancy and birth. Attending the exam gives him an opportunity to understand the emotional and physical changes that are taking place within your body.

INDICATIONS FOR CESAREAN SECTION

Cephalopelvic Disproportion

The most common reason for doing a cesarean section is called cephalopelvic disproportion. This means that your baby's head is too large to pass easily through your pelvis. Your pelvis may be unusually small or of an unusual shape, or your baby's head may be particularly large. Sometimes your doctor is able to predict a pelvic problem when making the internal examination at the beginning of your pregnancy. But most of the time, it is hard to tell if a disproportion exists until the end of the pregnancy or until labor is well under way.

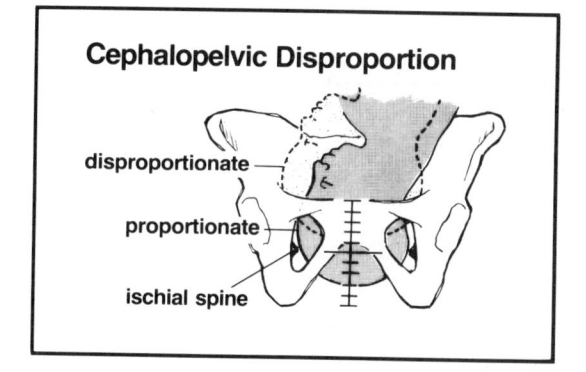

Malpresentation

Malpresentation means that a part of the baby other than his head is presented first. When the baby lies horizontally in the uterus, vaginal birth is impossible and a cesarean is always called for. In the breech presentation (see page 18), the buttocks or feet, instead of the head, are presented first. There are several kinds of breech presentations, but breech delivery always carries an increased risk of injury to the child. This is particularly true when the mother is over the age of thirty-five or the infant is large.

Poor Flexion

Even though your baby may be presented head first, if his chin is not flexed on his chest so that the back of his head comes first, complications may occur. A poorly flexed baby can result in an extremely difficult labor and in certain circumstances may be an indication for a cesarean.

Fetal Distress

During labor, those caring for you will always be aware of two lives: yours and your baby's. Throughout your labor they will be listening to your baby's heart tones. They indicate how he is responding to the rigors of labor and may signal a decrease in oxygen supply from the placenta to the fetus. If at any time your baby's heart tones indicate distress, a cesarean section may be the fastest way to accomplish safe delivery.

Prolapsed Cord

Uterine contractions may force the membranes of the placenta through an incompletely dilated cervix. If these membranes rupture early, the cord may prolapse, or extend past the presenting part. Once the cord is out of the uterus, and especially when out of the vagina, the blood and oxygen supply to your baby is obstructed and delivery must take place immediately.

Placenta Abruptio

Placenta abruptio occurs if the placenta separates from the uterine wall before the baby is delivered. Your baby is cut off from her source of oxygen and may suffer brain damage or die unless delivered quickly.

Placenta Previa

Placenta previa occurs if the placenta is located either at or partially covering the opening of the cervix. If labor were allowed to progress, the placenta would be delivered before the baby, and the life-giving oxygen supply to your baby would be cut off with disastrous consequences.

Prolonged Labor

If for any reason labor is considerably prolonged, a cesarean section will be considered. Patients are usually not permitted to labor longer than twenty-four hours if dilatation does not progress.

Other Reasons

1. If maternal distress is brought on by toxemia or hypertension.
2. If vaginal infections, such as herpes, occur at the end of pregnancy and endanger the baby as he passes through the birth canal.
3. If an attempt at inducing labor through chemical or physical means fails.
4. If forceps are necessary but endanger the mother or baby.
5. If the pregnancy is progressing beyond the forty-second or forty-third week.
6. If there is blood incompatibility, such as Rh factor.
7. If the mother is diagnosed as having diabetes mellitus.
8. If the mother has experienced a previous cesarean section. The possibility of a vaginal birth depends on many factors, such as the reason for the previous cesarean, the size of the baby in relation to the mother's pelvis, and the type of incision. If your last baby was delivered by cesarean because of the small size and shape of your pelvis and the large size of your child, and if this baby is also considered large for your pelvis, you probably should expect another cesarean childbirth.

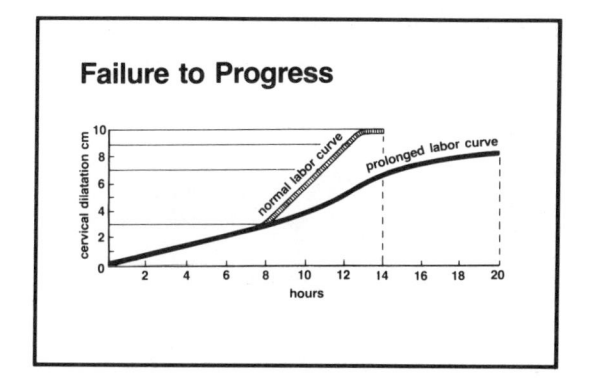

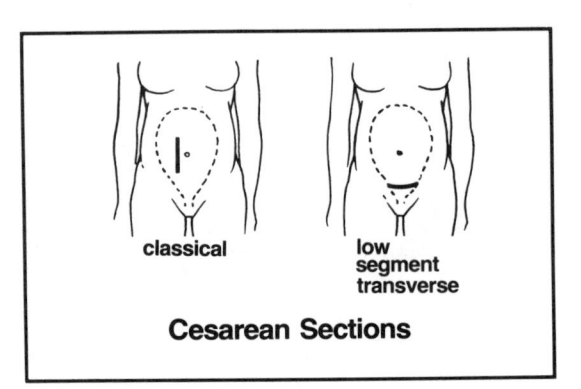

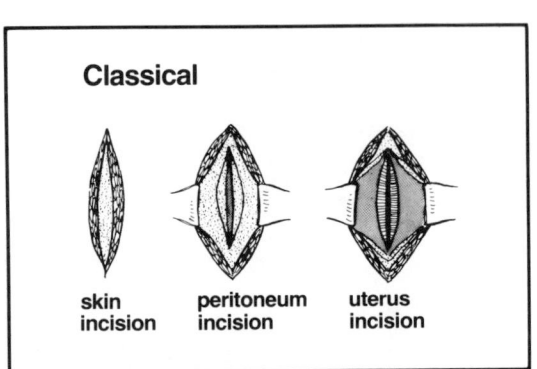

TYPES OF CESAREAN SECTIONS

Whether you know ahead of time that you will experience a cesarean, or whether the need arises during labor and an emergency cesarean is indicated, it is important that you be prepared and informed. First of all, you need to know that there are two types of cesarean section: the classical section and the low segment transverse cesarean. Surgery usually takes one to one and a half hours total, although your baby will be delivered within the first five to fifteen minutes. The remainder of the time is required to repair the incisions in your uterus and abdominal wall.

Classical

The classical cesarean section, used less commonly now, is indicated either when the baby's lie is totally abnormal or with a total placenta previa. An incision approximately five inches long is made from above the pubis to below the navel through the skin, abdominal muscle covering, and the muscles themselves. The loose covering membrane, called the peritoneum, is cut to expose the uterus. A four-inch vertical incision opens the uterus. The membranes are then ruptured and the hand of the doctor is inserted through the uterine incision to grasp either the head or one or both feet of your baby. The cord is cut and your baby is handed to an assistant. Shortly after delivery, your uterus contracts and bleeding usually ceases. The placenta and membranes separate spontaneously or are removed manually and are delivered through the incision. The uterine opening is then sewn closed in three layers: the uterus, peritoneum, and abdominal skin.

Low Segment Transverse (Bikini Incision)

The low segment transverse cesarean is one in which an incision is made just above your pubic hairline. The first incision opens the exterior skin of the abdomen and goes through the fat and muscle layers. The peritoneum is cut to expose the lower segment of your uterus. A small incision is made and then widened to about four inches. The surgeon puts his hand into your uterus to lift your baby's head, while an assistant presses the top of the uterus to help expel your baby. Sometimes it is necessary to extract the head with forceps. The membranes and placenta are then separated and delivered. The uterine incision is closed, followed by the closing of the peritoneum and the abdominal skin. The low segment incision is preferable because the incision is made in a section of the uterus that does not contract during labor. Blood loss is less, infection rate is lower, and the possibility of rupture of the scar in future births is reduced.

ANESTHESIA

Ask your anesthesiologist about the options in anesthesia and the benefits and risks of each. There are two types of anesthesia: general anesthesia, which allows you to be asleep during delivery; and spinal anesthesia, which allows you to be awake but have no feeling in your lower body. The type of anesthesia you receive depends on a number of things: the reason for your cesarean; whether it is an emergency or elective procedure; the size and position of your baby; your medical history; and your preference.

General

If you plan to be asleep during the cesarean, general anesthesia is used. An anesthesiologist gives you a medication, most likely sodium pentothal, which induces sleep within fifteen to twenty seconds. After you are asleep, a muscle relaxant and possibly nitrous oxide is administered by mask. Your progress will be continually monitored. When you are sufficiently sedated, surgery begins and your baby is born within minutes. As surgery is completed, medication is reduced, and you wake up as you go to the recovery room.

Saddle/Epidural

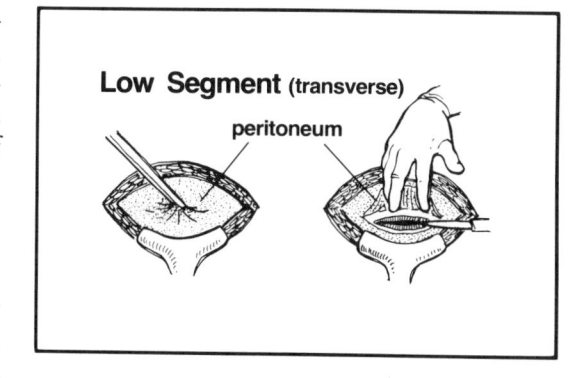

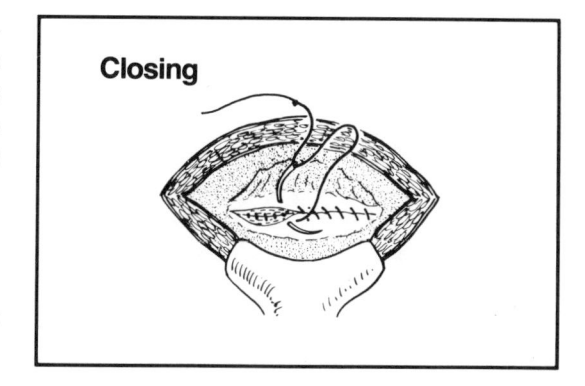

If you wish to be awake during your cesarean, you are given a spinal or saddle block so that you have no feeling in your lower body. You are asked to lie on your side, to curl your back and separate your vertebrae. Your skin is scrubbed and a small local injection given to numb the area. After this, a needle is inserted in your lower back, either into the spine itself or into the epidural space next to the spine, and medication similar to Novocain is given. The medication deadens the nerves from just above your navel down to your toes, and in a few minutes you have no sensation in your lower extremities.

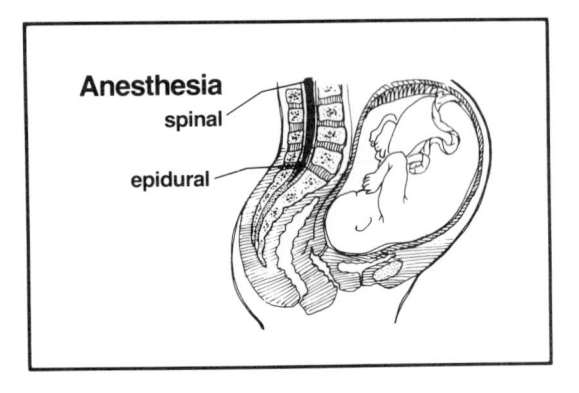

ESTABLISHING DUE DATE

One of the advantages of a nonemergency cesarean section is that you may participate in choosing your delivery date. Tests are often used to determine your baby's maturity. In the early weeks of pregnancy, your due date was estimated by determining the size of the uterus, the date fetal movements were first perceived, and the date at which the uterus reached the level of the navel. A much more accurate method for determining the baby's maturity is by analyzing a small quantity of amniotic fluid obtained through a procedure called amniocentesis. A small needle is inserted into the amniotic sac to obtain this fluid. An analysis of the fluid measures the lung maturity of your baby by comparing the ratio of lecithin to sphingomyelin present. These build up in the amniotic fluid from the baby's lungs in gradually increasing amounts with a marked increase after the thirty-fourth week.

Measuring the diameter of your baby's head with ultrasound can also help predict his growth and therefore set an estimated due date. Ultrasound determines the precise location and size of your baby's head, body, legs, arms, chest and, most importantly, placenta. Sound waves that are converted to images on a TV screen can be seen immediately and recorded by taking a picture of the screen.

PREOPERATIVE PROCEDURES

You will want to check into the hospital the night before your scheduled cesarean so you can take care of preoperative procedures such as admission forms, weighing in, blood and urine samples, and a complete physical examination.

Labor Room

Even though you have a set date for your cesarean delivery, you may spontaneously begin labor before it. If your membranes rupture or if your uterine contractions come with increasing intensity every five minutes, you should contact your doctor immediately and then go to the hospital. Do not eat or drink anything. You will be prepared for surgery upon arrival.

If you are in active labor, blood and urine samples will be taken as you enter the hospital. You will also be weighed and have your blood pressure and pulse taken. Then you will be given an enema. Your abdomen will be shaved and scrubbed with an antiseptic. While you wait for surgery to begin, you should use deep breathing and relaxation to control your contractions.

Your temperature and blood pressure and your baby's heartbeat will be checked. Your watch, earrings, rings, and anything else that can come off are given to the nurse for safekeeping. You may wear your glasses or contact lenses if you plan to be awake. About thirty minutes before your cesarean is scheduled, your anesthesiologist will help take you to the delivery room on a rolling stretcher.

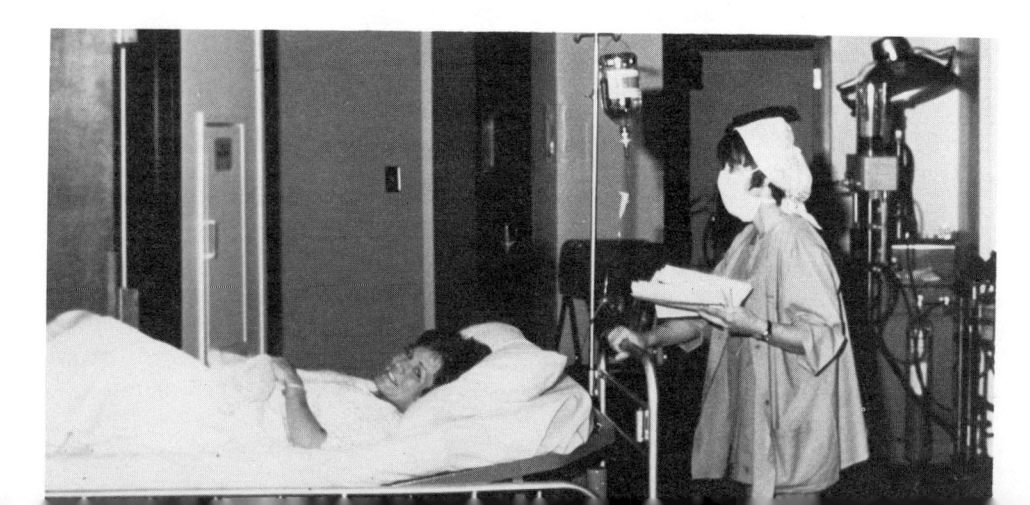

Operating Room

In the operating room, you will be surrounded by a medical team that will be responsible for both your safety and your baby's healthy delivery. Your obstetrician will be assisted by another doctor. Your pediatrician will be there to care for your newborn from the first moments after birth. Your anesthesiologist will assume the vital role of controlling the level of anesthesia. Nurses will be present to assist and participate with you in the miracle of your baby's birth.

An intravenous solution will be started in the IV previously put in your arm. This will provide water and any medication you might need throughout and after the operation. A catheter will be inserted into your bladder to keep it empty. Because the bladder is close to the uterus, it must be kept empty to help delivery and to prevent injury during surgery.

If your baby's father is to be with you during delivery, he will now be called in and will remain by your side. He will be able to give you constant comfort and encouragement and to remind you to relax and breathe deeply. You will be draped with sterile sheets. A screen will be placed across your shoulders. Although you cannot see over this screen, the baby's father will be able to describe the progress of the delivery of your baby.

CESAREAN SURGERY

Incisions

If you have had a previous cesarean section, surgery will begin with an incision in the abdominal wall at the old scar line. The old scar tissue is removed. The incision goes through the fat layer. Your bladder and abdominal contents are moved to the side. Another incision is made into the membrane covering the abdomen and your uterus is exposed. An incision is then made into the low, noncontracting part of the uterus. The incision through the uterus exposes the amniotic membranes, which are then ruptured.

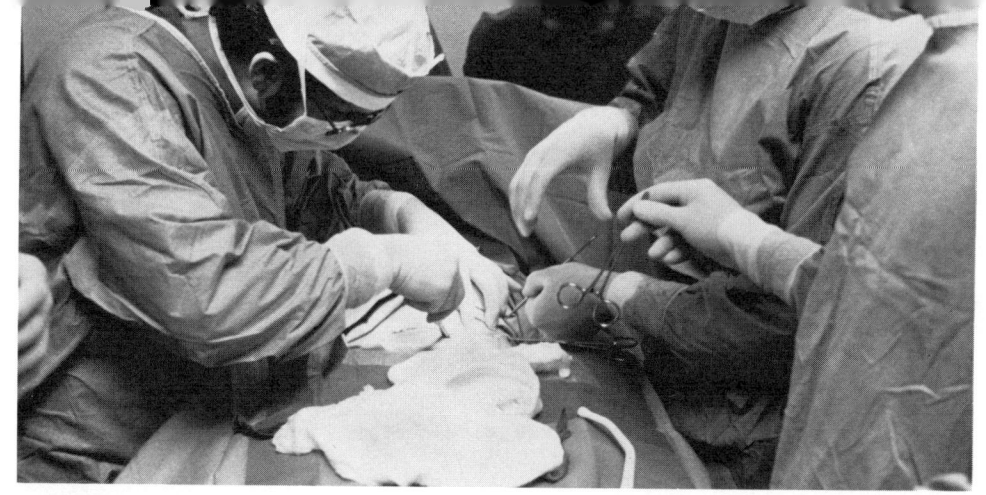

Birth

Your doctor will reach in with his hand and gently draw the baby out. Since your baby may be tightly wedged, your doctor may apply pressure below the pubic bone. His assistant will push down on your upper abdomen to help expel the baby.

Once your baby is born, your doctor will clamp the umbilical cord. He will hand the baby to the waiting pediatrician, who will suction the mucus out of the baby's mouth.

Repair of Incision

After the placenta is delivered, the uterine incision is closed, the inner halves of the cut edges are sutured, and the outer edges of the uterus are brought together. The membranes of the peritoneum covering the abdomen are closed after any blood that may have escaped into the pelvic cavity has been sponged out. The abdominal incision is then closed with special skin clips.

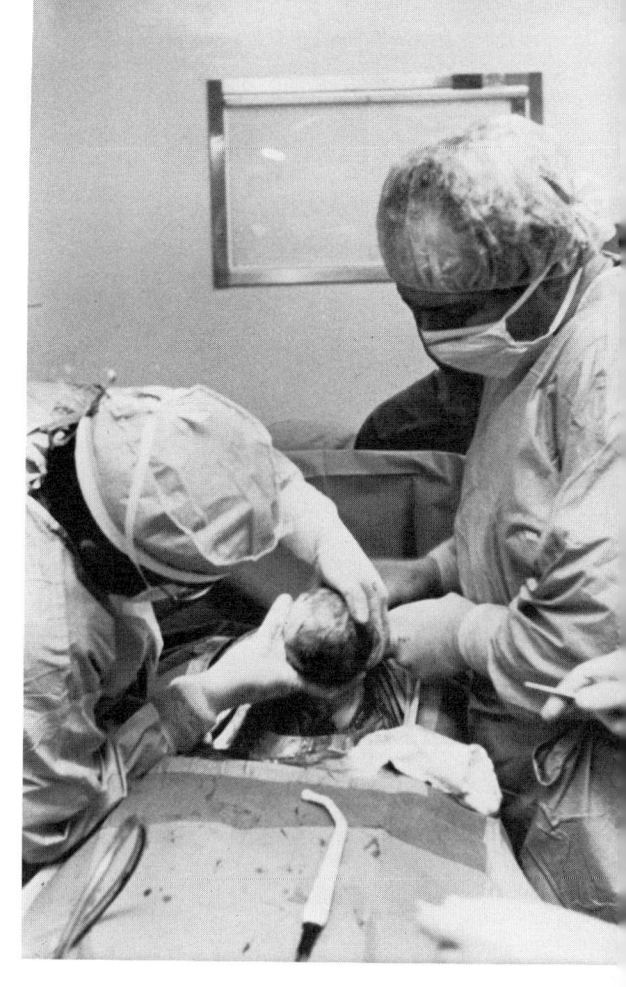

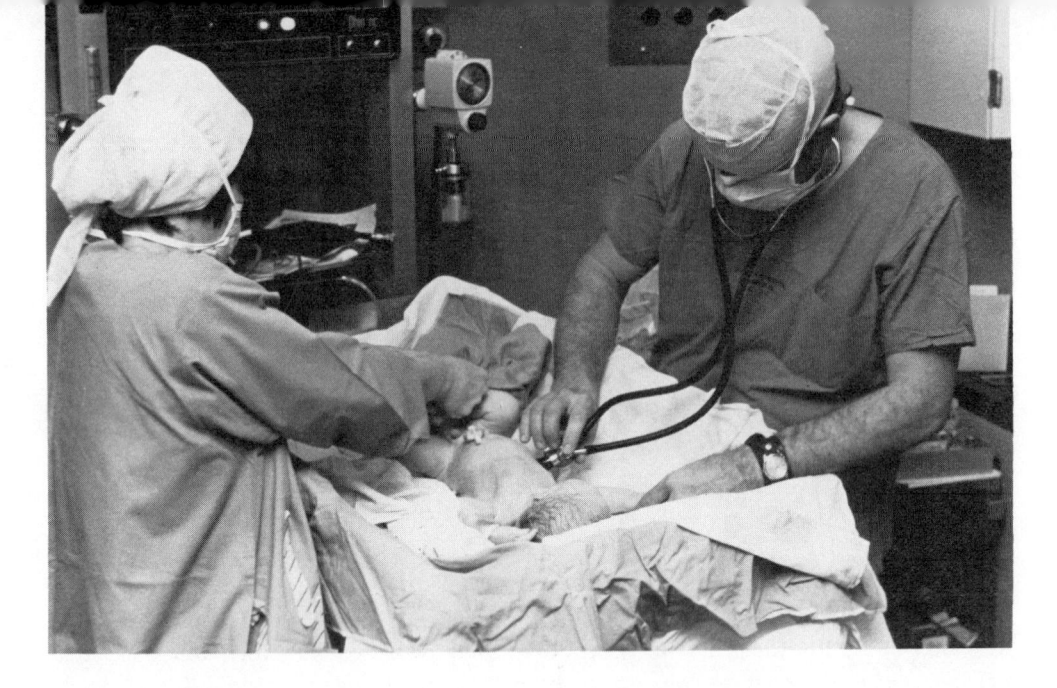

Pediatric Care

It is advisable to have a physician responsible for your baby at birth, since infants born by cesarean section may have respiratory problems. An infant born by cesarean section misses the pressure of passage through the birth canal which, in vaginal birth, activates all of his systems and expels fluid and mucus from his respiratory system.

Your pediatrician will quickly place your baby in a special unit to maintain his temperature and administer oxygen if needed. He will make a thorough examination, suction amniotic fluid and mucus from your baby's mouth, and listen to his heartbeat and breathing. Your baby may be able to be with you immediately after birth or, for many reasons, your baby may be taken to the nursery for observation.

Recovery Room

You will be taken to the recovery room following your cesarean birth and given medication to ease any pain you may be experiencing. The nurse will check your pulse, blood pressure, temperature, and respiration to be sure that your systems have stabilized and are responding normally. You will be kept under observation in case there is excessive bleeding from the vagina or the incision. You will remain in the recovery room until you can move both legs, and your baby's father will be allowed to be with you. He can give you valuable support, comfort, and encouragement.

You will have vaginal bleeding just as in a vaginal delivery. The hospital will provide belts and sanitary napkins. If the metal clasp on the sanitary belt rubs, you can attach the pads directly to your underwear by an adhesive strip, or place an extra pad under the clasp. The nurses will constantly check the quantity and quality of the vaginal flow.

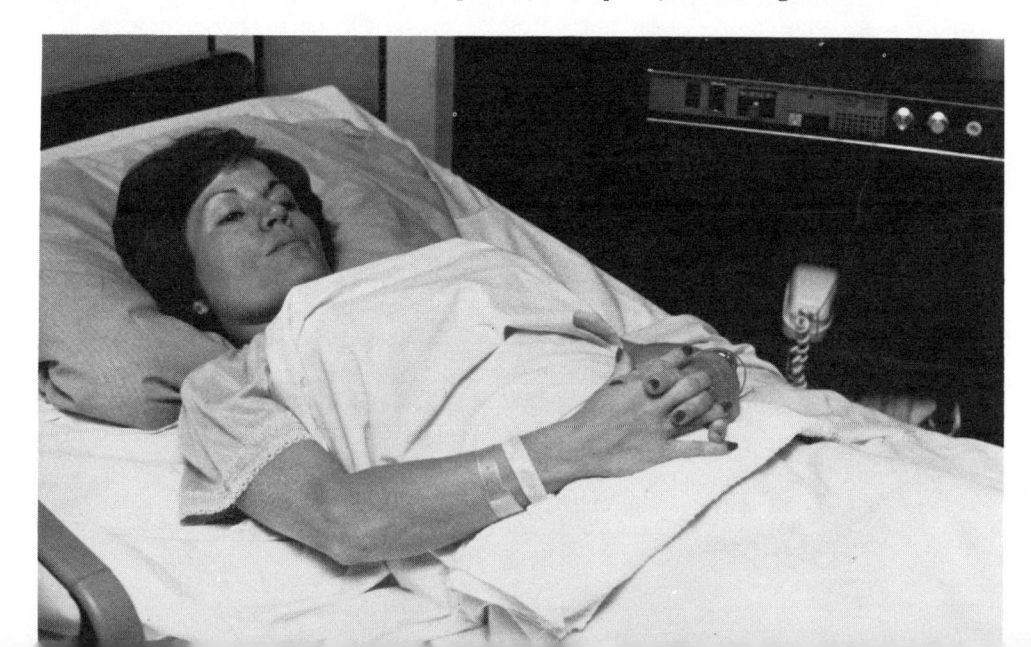

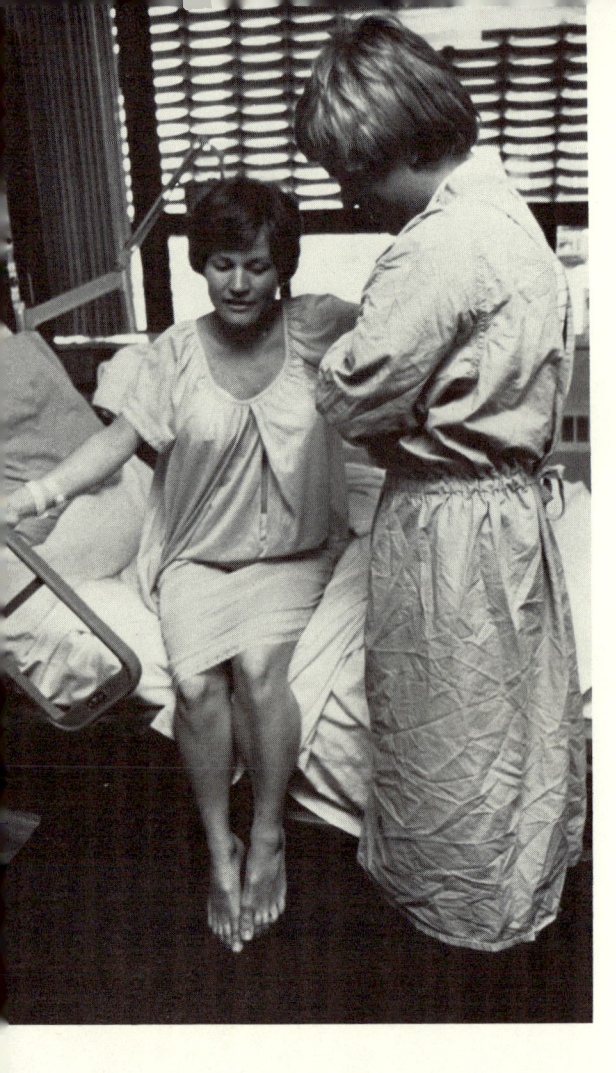

POSTPARTUM

Recovery

After the recovery room, you will be taken to your room on the maternity floor. The nurse will tell you that moving is the best cure for postsurgical pain and that the more you move about, the sooner you will feel better. Move your feet and ankles, wiggle your toes, and stretch your arms.

Learning to splint your incision will decrease the pain when you move. Interlace your fingers and place your hands, palms down, over the incision to support it. Press firmly but gently, take a deep breath two to three times, and cough deeply once. This can also be done by using a pillow held against the incision with your arms wrapped around it to apply gentle pressure.

The average hospital stay is six to seven days. You will be asked to get up and walk around the day after your cesarean and will be encouraged to do so several times a day. You will probably need help taking your first few steps. Although you will be uncomfortable, the sooner you begin moving the sooner you will recover. To get out of bed, crank the head of your bed as high as it will go and inch your body to the side of the bed. As you slowly swing your feet to the side, have someone help you sit up. Dangle your feet until they feel comfortable. When you are ready, have someone help you to stand and straighten up very gradually. Take a deep breath and relax. It is common to feel as if your incision will open. To counter this feeling, carefully splint your incision with your hands. Stand as straight as possible and breathe deeply. Each step will get easier.

The catheter inserted during the operation will be left in place until you are able to walk to the bathroom by yourself. After it is removed, have someone help you to the toilet. Be sure to keep track of your urine volume. The nurse will remind you that it is important to drink plenty of fluids to avoid becoming dehydrated. This is especially important if you are breast-feeding.

Blood and air collected under the diaphragm may cause pain in your shoulders; there are nerve connections between the diaphragm and shoulder. You may have abdominal discomfort for two or three days after surgery. Your incision should heal in two to three

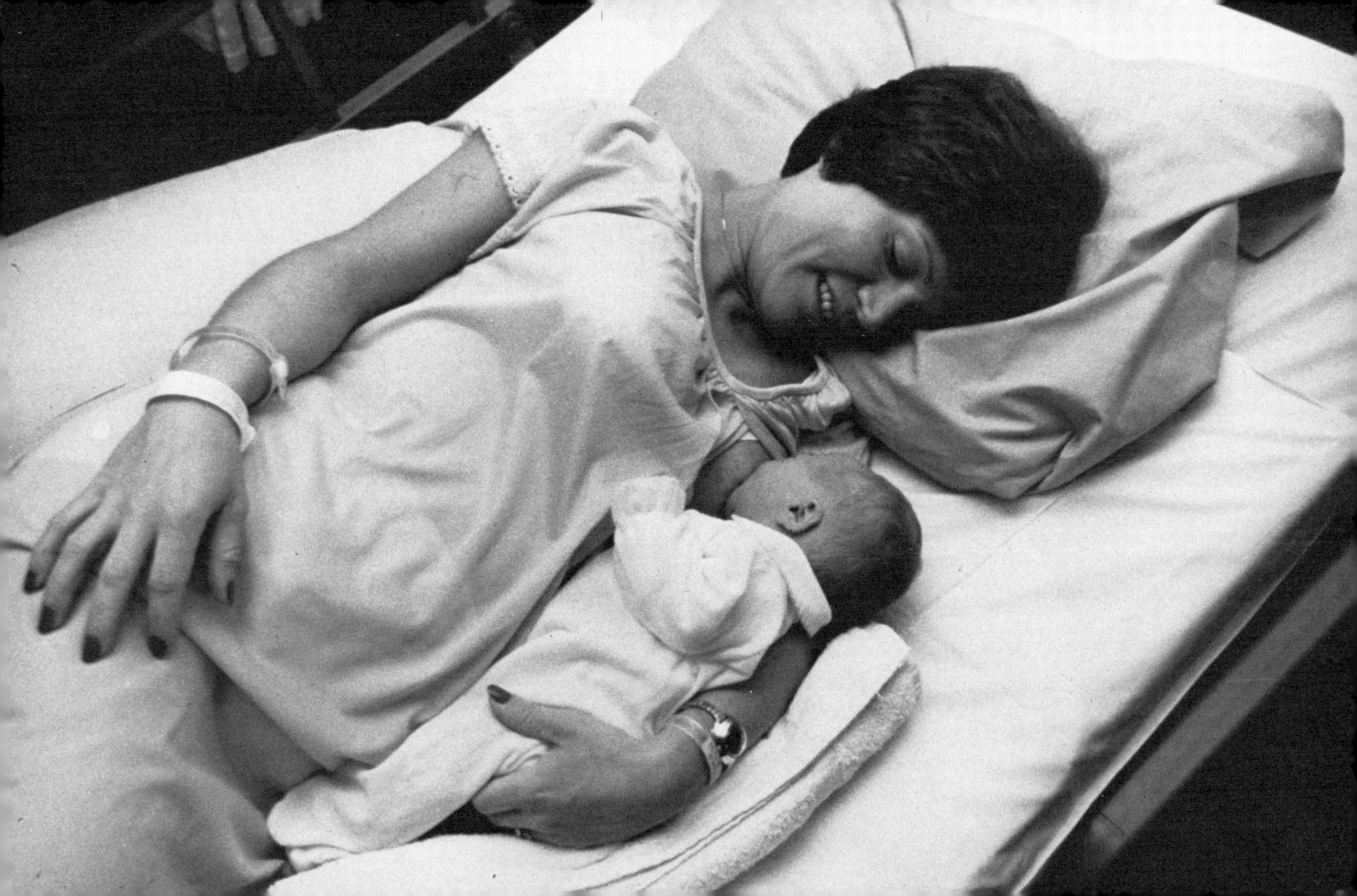

weeks and you can expect to feel quite well by a week to ten days after surgery. By the third day your intestinal tract begins to function again and you may experience sharp gas pains. This can be alleviated by having the nurse insert a flexible tube into your rectum to help you pass gas. Carbonated drinks, coffee, and tea make gas worse and should be avoided at this time.

Your doctor will visit you during your hospitalization and will want to check your incision. He will change the dressing, which is a woven, stretchy fabric applied with adhesive to the abdomen. It gives you support and a secure feeling.

Your skin clips or stitches will be removed before you go home. It is important to look at the incision since the fear of the unknown is worse than the reality. It is normal for the scar to be itchy, or numb, and to pull and ooze a bit.

Postpartum exercises are important in recovering from a cesarean birth. A well-rounded program of exercise should begin as soon as possible.

Breast-feeding

Mothers who have had a cesarean birth are able to breast-feed successfully, even though getting started may be slower than usual. Since breast-feeding stimulates the uterus to contract and return to its normal state, it is an important part of recovery.

Pick a position that is comfortable. Sit up and support your baby's head with your arm and tuck a pillow under your baby's body. Place his mouth at the level of your nipple and allow your breast to touch his cheek to encourage his rooting reflex.

Nursing while lying down may be more comfortable and can help assure you of the rest and relaxation you need. Lie on your side and hold your baby facing you. Place your baby's mouth close to your nipple and allow it to touch his cheek, again prompting the rooting reflex. By trying different nursing positions you can find what works best for you and your baby. Although milk does not flow immediately after birth, you will be giving your baby valuable colostrum, which passes on some of your immunities. Many babies do not show interest in feeding for a few days; remember that it takes time to learn together.

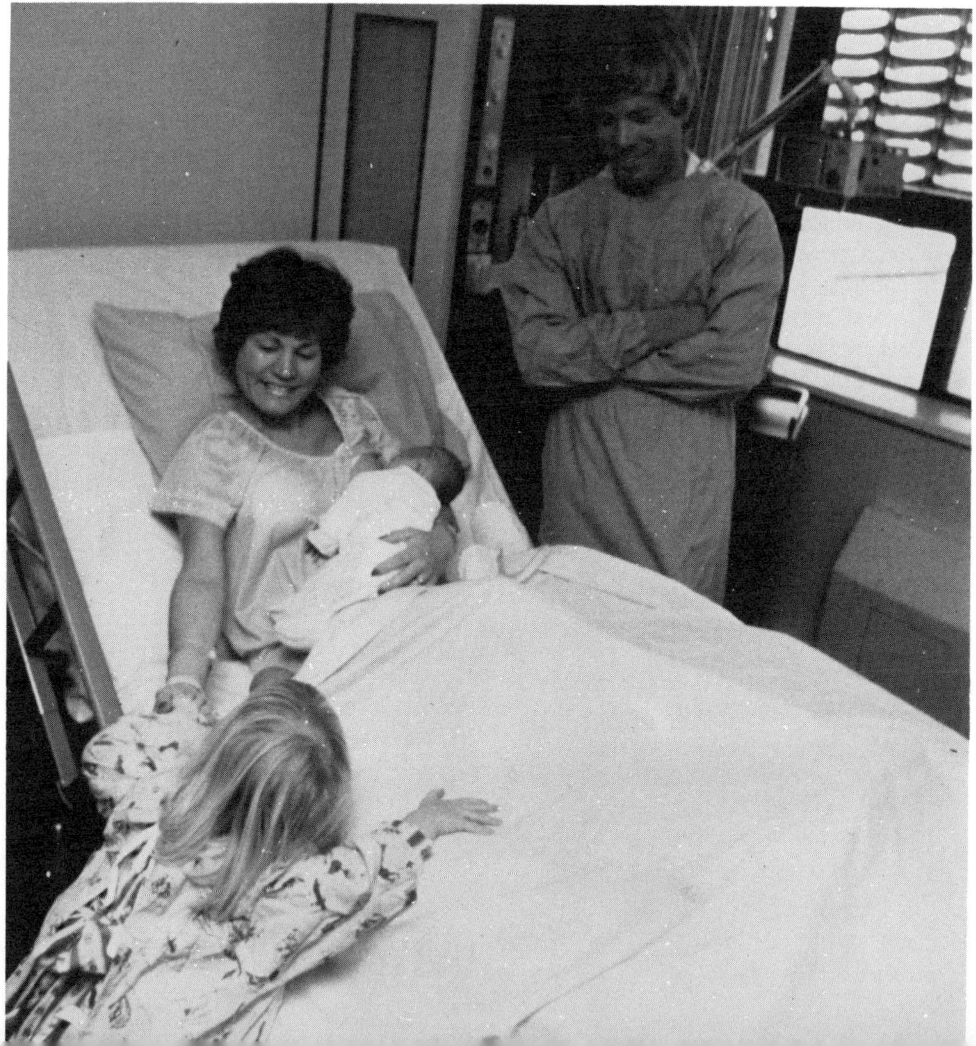

Emotions

After any childbirth it is common for parents to experience feelings of depression, helplessness, guilt, ambivalence, and panic. These feelings seem to be even more pronounced after a cesarean childbirth. It is common to feel anger, resentment, and inadequacy and to experience a loss of self-esteem. At this time, it will be important for you to express your feelings and concerns. Communication will help you and your baby's father develop a mutual understanding and empathy with each other. No person understands better than those who have experienced a cesarean birth themselves. There are local cesarean support groups you can contact immediately after your experience to talk about your physical and emotional concerns.

Because you will be able to participate in the planning of your baby's birth and will be prepared for what will happen, you should feel that you have some control over your life. Your cesarean childbirth can be a joyful experience in which you can focus not on the fear of surgery, but on the joy of birth. As an active participant, you will develop bonds that will give your baby a first lesson in giving and accepting love.

13.

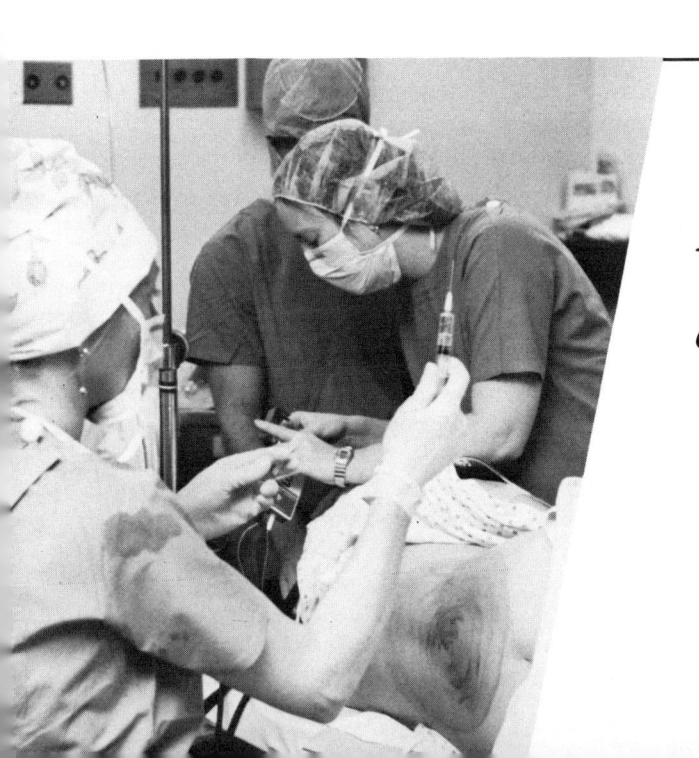

Medical Intervention and Anesthetics

Interventions are obstetrical procedures that, although not necessary in the routine process of labor and delivery, do help your birthing attendant by providing information about your baby, yourself, or the quality of your labor. Some of them allow problem situations to be identified and dealt with early. Those persons who have needed and received special care are grateful for advanced techniques and technology. Induction, ultrasound, fetal monitoring, anesthesia, cesarean section, and the development of special skills in treating newborns (called neonatology) have increased both the quantity and the quality of life for premature babies and full-term babies born with problems or complications.

Although there has been legitimate protest against obstetrical care that treats all pregnancies and births as high-risk cases, the availability of advanced techniques and technology has saved or enhanced many lives. But each procedure carries with it some drawbacks. It is to your advantage to understand what interventions are available, how and when they can be of benefit to you and your baby, and what disadvantages they carry with them.

INTERVENTIONS

Intravenous (IV) Fluids

Procedure. If the mother needs extra fluids or sustenance during labor, a needle is placed in a vein in the back of her hand or in her arm. Attached to the needle is a tube leading to a bottle of, for example, dextrose and water, which will drip continually into her vein. If, for any reason, the mother's condition becomes distressed, the needle is instantly available for medications.

Benefits. If the mother experiences a long, fatiguing labor, the IV provides her with some fluid and some energy. If she needs medication, her attendants have immediate access to her vein. If her labor becomes ineffective, the IV setup is readily available to augment it with hormones.

Drawbacks. In a normal labor a mother can receive her liquids and energy from other sources and will probably have no need for intravenous medications or anesthetics, so it is an unnecessary procedure that restricts her movement and walking.

Stripping the Membranes

Procedure. Before labor, during a pelvic examination, the attendant can "speed things up" or induce labor by inserting a finger between the membranes and the cervix and separating the membranes from the lower part of the uterus. This procedure must be performed when the cervix is softening and effacing. Usually, the mother will experience a small amount of bloody mucous discharge.

Benefits. If, after assessing the cervix and the estimated due date, the baby is evaluated to be overdue, this procedure may begin labor.

Drawbacks. If the cervix is not ready, the process will be ineffective.

Induction and Augmentation

Procedure. Pitocin or some other synthetic hormone is given to the mother, either intravenously or by mouth, to generate the uterine contractions and cause them to increase in strength and frequency. This technique can either be used to start labor (induction), or it is used during labor if the contractions have become irregular, inconsistent, or weak (augmentation).

Benefits. This technique is indicated if the membranes have ruptured and labor has failed to begin. If the mother is distressed by toxemia or diabetes, and it is medically sound to deliver the baby before birth begins naturally, or if, during labor, the uterine contractions become ineffectual, induction or augmentation may be called for.

Drawbacks. Induced contractions are often more intense and difficult for the laboring woman to control. The stress and medications have serious side effects for both mother and baby and the mother must be closely observed. Pitocin can cause a drop in her blood pressure, increased heart rate, and water retention. It can cause prolonged contractions and even rupture of the uterus. Pitocin can cause changes in the baby's heart rate and a decrease in his oxygen supply. There are also some studies that associate pitocin with jaundice in the newborn.

Enema and Shaving

Procedure. Traditionally a woman in labor entering a hospital is given an enema and her pubic hair is shaved. The enema is given to clear the colon of residual feces and shaving the pubic hair is done to facilitate repair of the episiotomy site.

Benefits. Although the diarrhea of prelabor and early labor is nature's way of emptying the bowels in preparation for labor and delivery, if a woman has an enema, she may feel freer to push without having to worry about the possibility of a bowel movement during delivery.

Drawbacks. Enemas are not risky, but they may be undignified and contrived at a time when a woman is trying to retain her dignity and self-esteem. Some women choose to give themselves a Fleet's enema early in labor. Although a shave is not risky, it can be irritating both when the area is shaved and when the hair is growing back. Recent research has shown that there is no difference in the infection rate for shaved and unshaved women who have had an episiotomy repair.

Episiotomy

Procedure. During the part of delivery just before the baby's head emerges, the doctor or birth attendant makes a surgical incision from the mother's vagina toward the rectum. This incision may be either a straight line back to the rectum or angled to the right or left. Episiotomies may have become a routine part of American birthing because a woman in the traditional but unnatural position, lying on her back on a delivery table with her legs up in stirrups, puts the pressure of her baby's head on her perineum rather than on the vaginal outlet. This makes tearing of the perineum, especially with the first baby, almost inevitable. This position, combined with the routine use of a pudendal block, which anesthetizes the pelvic floor and takes away the natural stretching sensations that cause a woman to quit pushing at the crowning of her baby's head, makes an episiotomy almost inevitable. A woman who pushes in a sitting or side-lying position who has not had a pudendal, who is able to stop pushing as the baby's head emerges and who has a supportive physician who does not give routine episiotomies is more likely to deliver without an episiotomy.

Benefits. In the days before episiotomies, some women suffered gross tearing and infection. When a baby's head is especially large or the mother's pushing efforts uncontrolled, an episiotomy provides a measure of control to avoid tearing the perineal tissues. Repair of a tear may be quite difficult and painful for the mother, whereas repair of the surgical incision is easier and quicker. Episiotomies are always necessary when forceps or vacuum extraction is performed.

Drawbacks. Most women who have episiotomies experience a great deal of postpartum pain in the healing of the incision. This pain may inhibit the ability to breast-feed and may interfere with the natural process of bonding. There is also some indication that the episiotomy adds to the discomfort and fear of resuming intercourse and may contribute to poor postpartum sexual adjustments.

External Electronic Fetal Monitor

Procedure. Electronic fetal monitoring (EFM) is probably one of the most commonly used procedures to evaluate the effect of your contractions on the baby during labor. The external monitor measures the baby's heart rate and the quality and rate of contractions from outside the mother's body. An elasticized or rubberized belt with two small round sensors is placed around your abdomen. One is an ultrasound device to measure the baby's heart rate and how it reacts with each contraction; the other is a pressure-sensitive device to measure the intensity, length, and interval of every contraction. The measurements are printed together on graph paper, indicating the relationship between your contractions and your baby's heartbeat.

Benefits. Medical staff who work with the EFM are able to assess the quality and frequency of your contractions. Your baby's general physical state can be evaluated by observing his heart rate in relation to the contractions. Most important, fetal distress can be picked up early in labor and early intervention techniques can be started. When anesthetics or induced labor are used, the birthing attendant can assess their effect on both the baby and the contractions. Medical staff who support the use of the EFM say that when complications occur in labor, it allows them to intervene at an earlier stage and deliver healthier and more viable babies. Many coaches and even women say that the EFM helps them assess the beginning, peak, and end of the contractions.

Drawbacks. Several studies have shown that a medical staff well trained in using a stethoscope to listen to the quality of the baby's heartbeat, and who stay with the woman throughout her labor, giving her constant personal attention, can deliver as healthy a baby as if they had used the EFM. This type of care has the added advantage of giving the emotional support a woman needs during labor and delivery. With the EFM the medical staff may not give the woman as much emotional support as they might if they were not using it. It is also possible for the machine to break down. The belt is restrictive and uncomfortable. If the mother is forced to lie on her back for the monitor it may slow her labor and cut down oxygen to her baby.

Internal Electronic Fetal Monitor

Procedure. The internal monitor gives essentially the same information as the external EFM. The internal monitor has two tubes that are inserted through the vagina to the scalp of the baby. At the end of one of the tubes is an electrode that is attached to the baby's scalp and picks up and records your baby's heart rate. The other has a pressure-sensitive device that measures and records intrauterine pressure with each contraction.

Benefits. The internal EFM is more accurate than the external one. It is more comfortable for the mother, since she does not have the restrictive belt around her abdomen and she may move around more freely.

Drawbacks. With the internal monitor there is a greater chance of infection for both mother and baby. The membranes must be ruptured to insert the EFM, which can change the quality of your labor. Although the mother is freer to move around with the internal monitor, her movements are still somewhat restricted.

Forceps

Procedure. Forceps are an instrument designed to fit around the baby's head much like a football helmet. They are applied to both sides of the baby's head to assist in the rotation of the head during birth. There are high, medium, and low uses of forceps. The high and medium positions, in which the physician goes up into the mother's body to deliver the baby, are almost never used today and are the source of ancient tales of horror and deformity. Cesarean section has taken the place of this use of the forceps. Today, low forceps are used simply to help guide the baby's head out or to help turn it for an easier delivery.

Benefits. Forceps can help when the mother is experiencing difficulty in her last pushing efforts because of the size of the head or the position of the presenting part (usually posterior). Forceps are also indicated when the mother has been anesthetized and cannot actively push her baby out. If the baby is premature, forceps can protect its head from prolonged pressure in the birth canal.

Drawbacks. When forceps are used, the mother feels more painful sensations and she must always have an episiotomy. Forceps may bruise the soft tissues of the baby's face or head.

Extractor

Procedure. An extractor is a device applied to the baby's head by creating a vacuum between the baby's scalp and the cap of the extractor. The baby is then carefully and slowly pulled out by the birth attendant. The extractor may be used in place of low forceps for delivery.

Benefits. The extractor can help turn the baby's head, deliver the baby's head, hasten delivery, and protect the baby from prolonged pressure in the birth canal.

Drawbacks. Use of the extractor may result in swollen tissues of the baby's scalp.

ANESTHETICS AND PAIN RELIEVERS

Anesthetics were first introduced in the days of Queen Victoria. Their use soon spread to the general populace and, up until recent times, anesthesia was a traditional and routine part of childbirth. However, parents who wished to be awake and aware during the birth of their babies began to question their use. Research has uncovered more and more evidence that the routine use of anesthesia and pain relievers in a normal labor and delivery is questionable. There is no drug that does not have some side effects for either the mother or the baby. And recent research has turned up not only short-term effects, but more important, long-term ones. Today, a growing number of people in the medical community are reevaluating the routine use of medications in uncomplicated births. At the same time, educated parents now go into a normal labor and delivery prepared for some discomfort as a common and natural part of birth.

Just as important, educated parents are aware that although drugs given to a mother during labor or delivery do affect a baby, there are certain circumstances in which medications are necessary for the well-being of both mother and baby. Fetal distress, maternal distress, or prolonged or abnormal labor are all indications for obstetrical intervention, which will usually call for some kind of medication.

Whether this is your first or your fourth baby, you cannot know beforehand what kind of a labor and delivery you will have. But you do know that you want a healthy baby and a healthy outcome above all. So you should be aware not only of the problems and complications that might arise in your labor, but also of the common kinds of medications and their benefits and risks, should the need for any of them arise. It is important that you talk to your doctor or medical caregiver *before* labor and delivery to discuss his or her philosophy (when they use medications) and preferences (what medications they prefer).

Medications for childbirth fall into five major groups: sedatives (which calm and relax the mother), tranquilizers (which relieve tension), analgesics (pain relievers), regional anesthetics (which deaden specific areas), and general anesthetics (which result in complete unconsciousness).

Sedatives

Sedatives, such as barbiturates, are given early in labor to calm the mother.

Benefits. Should a mother be extremely tense in early labor, a sedative may help her relax and perhaps rest.

Drawbacks. Given too soon, sedatives can slow your labor. They can cause drowsiness. You may become disoriented and out of control. A buildup of sedatives in your baby's system can cause respiratory distress, poor responsiveness, and poor sucking abilities after birth.

Tranquilizers

Tranquilizers such as Vistaril, Valium, Librium, and Miltown are usually given later in labor.

Benefits. Tranquilizers can help relieve anxiety in a very tense mother. Some can help reduce feelings of nausea.

Drawbacks. Tranquilizers may produce a change in your blood pressure and cause drowsiness, dizziness, and confusion. They may also produce changes in your baby's heart rate, low body temperature, and poor muscle tone at birth.

Analgesics

Analgesics, such as Demerol and morphine, may be given to the mother in the active phase of labor to reduce pain. Analgesics work in the brain to alter the mother's perception of pain.

Benefits. Analgesics can reduce the mother's perception of pain without causing her to lose consciousness.

Drawbacks. Analgesics may cause a drop in your blood pressure. They may cause you to feel dizzy or nauseated, and they may make it difficult for you to concentrate on your relaxation and breathing techniques. If given too early, analgesics can alter your contraction patterns and slow your labor. They can cause problems in your baby's respiration and may depress his system and responses for some time after birth.

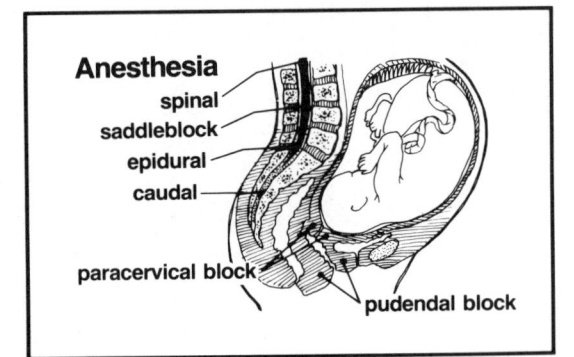

Regional Anesthetics

Anesthetics such as Novocain, Nesacaine, and Xylocaine are injected into nerve trunks, which lead to the areas to be numbed. There are several types of regional anesthetics that deaden the various areas affected by contractions and pressure areas as your baby moves through the birth canal. The major areas are the uterus, cervix, vagina, perineum, and pelvic floor.

PARACERVICAL BLOCK

The paracervical block anesthetizes only the uterus and cervix. It is injected into the nerve endings at both sides of the cervix. If given too early it may slow labor, so it is usually administered when the cervix is from four to nine centimeters dilated. Once the cervix is completely taken into the uterus, it can no longer be administered. The paracervical can take effect in just a few minutes and usually lasts from one to two hours.

Benefits. The paracervical takes effect immediately and gives relief.

Drawbacks. The paracervical is effective only about 80 percent of the time. It may take effect on one side and not the other, resulting in confusing sensations. When the paracervical wears off, the intensity of the contractions may be a sudden shock. It does not anesthetize the pelvic floor and another anesthetic is necessary for episiotomy repair.

Since the paracervical may require more medication than other types of regional anesthetics, it may result in more fetal absorption of the drug. The effects of a paracervical may cause the baby's heart rate to slow.

CAUDAL BLOCK

The caudal is a local anesthetic injected in the caudal canal at the base of the sacrum. The caudal procedure gives the mother relief in the uterus, the cervix, the vagina, the pelvic floor, and the perineum. It is usually given after five centimeters dilatation and takes fifteen to twenty minutes to take effect. It can last up to one and a half hours.

Benefits. Proponents of the caudal feel that its success rate is superior to that of the paracervical. It is longer lasting and requires less medication than the paracervical. It numbs the pelvic floor for any perineal procedures. The caudal may be given repeatedly through a catheter placed in the caudal canal, giving the woman continual comfort through her labor.

Drawbacks. The caudal may cause a drop in the mother's blood pressure, which, in turn, will cause a drop in the baby's heart rate. A woman with a caudal does not have the normal urge to push, thus necessitating more frequent use of forceps and episiotomy.

EPIDURAL BLOCK

The epidural is similar to the caudal. Placed in the lumbar spinal region, it affects the area between the waist and the knees. It is usually given after five centimeters dilatation and takes effect in ten to fifteen minutes.

Benefits. The epidural gives the mother complete comfort in the areas of her body affected by labor and delivery.

Drawbacks. Mothers who have epidurals lose their urge to push and forceps must be used in the birth of their babies. Forceps cause an episiotomy to be performed. Epidurals may also cause the mother's blood pressure to drop, resulting in a drop in her baby's heart rate.

SPINAL BLOCK

The spinal is injected into the lumbar area. It is usually given shortly before delivery. The spinal affects all the area from the breasts down to the toes. The effect is immediate and lasts about an hour.

Benefits. The spinal is effective when used for discomfort during delivery or when forceps are necessary. It is currently used by many modern physicians for cesarean births when the mother wishes to remain awake.

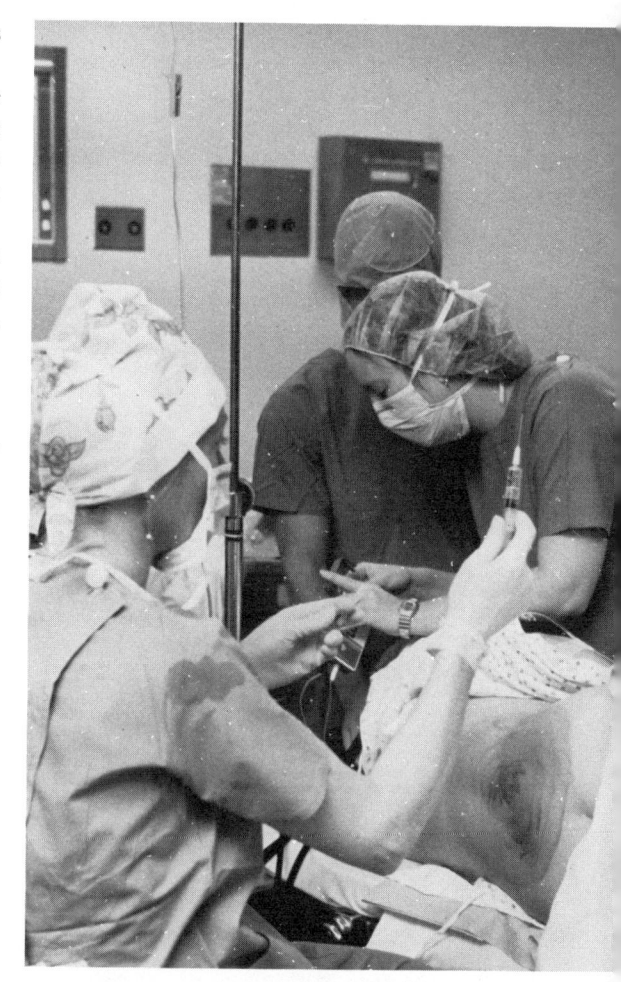

Drawbacks. The major disadvantage of the spinal is the "spinal headache" it produces. In addition, the mother's blood pressure may drop and she may experience difficulty in urinating after the birth of her baby. Again, the mother has no pushing sensation and the baby must be delivered by forceps.

SADDLE BLOCK

The saddle block is a type of spinal anesthesia in which the medication is injected into the vaginal canal fluid. It affects the area of the mother's body that would be in contact with a saddle: the inner thighs, genitals, and perineum.

Benefits. The saddle is quick to take effect and the mother does not lose feeling in her lower legs or toes.

Drawbacks. The mother may lose both sensation and movement. She may suffer from a spinal headache or lowered blood pressure.

PUDENDAL BLOCK

The pudendal block is a local anesthetic injected through the vagina into the pudendal nerves near the ischial spines. This type of anesthesia numbs the vagina and perineum and is used for the delivery and episiotomy repair. It is given before the birth of the baby. It takes effect in two to three minutes and lasts for one hour.

Benefits. The pudendal blocks sensation at the perineum for the birth and episiotomy.

Drawbacks. The pudendal block also numbs sensations during birth, allowing the mother to push without control, which can cause tearing of the perineal area. It may inhibit pushing by relaxing the muscles of the perineum. Although the risks to the baby are not known, it may cause depression of the baby's system.

LOCAL

Local anesthesia is injected directly into the perineum for the episiotomy or its repair.

Benefits. If an episiotomy is performed, the local anesthetizes the site.

Drawbacks. None documented, although some research indicates there may be some risk to the baby.

Scopalomine (Twilight Sleep)

Although the most common anesthetic of our grandmother's generation, twilight sleep is rarely used in modern obstetrics. Combined with morphine it provided mothers both sedation and a memory depressant.

Drawbacks. Scopalomine was intended to sedate the mother's pain and dull her memory. In actuality, it left a mother with a terrible nightmare quality of birth.

Scopalomine produces mothers who are unconscious, out of control, and dizzy with palpitations, depression, and respiratory distress. Since they are unconscious they are unable to witness their births. Their newborns are often born blue with great respiratory distress (they almost all have to be resuscitated after birth). Neither the mother nor the baby is able to function normally for some time after birth, resulting in mother/infant separation and difficulty in establishing successful breast-feeding patterns.

General Anesthetics

Agents such as ether or nitrous oxide may be given during birth when a need for immediate intervention calls for the mother's complete unconsciousness. This type of anesthesia depresses the nervous system to a point where the mother must be carefully monitored. Many hospitals today use general anesthesia only in emergency cesarean sections, preferring to use regional anesthesia so the mother may be awake during the birth of her baby.

Benefits. General anesthetics quickly produce complete unconsciousness when it is medically indicated.

Drawbacks. General anesthesia may bring contractions to a halt and depress the mother's system. It also causes newborn respiratory distress and depression. It may take the infant over a week to recover.

Assessing the Need for Anesthetics

Considering the research on the risks of medications, the modern medical staff does not want to give anesthetics if they are not needed. There are three major components your attendant considers in assessing when you need medication and what type of medication to give.

First, your caregiver evaluates the general conditions of your labor. How effective are your contractions? How big is your baby and what position is he in? What is your history of past labors?

Second, your attendant will monitor how well your baby is reacting to the contractions. If the baby shows distress, some sort of medical intervention will be considered. If your labor is not progressing at a normal rate and problems or complications are suspected, medical intervention will be considered.

Third, your caregiver will assess how well you are handling your contractions. If you seem in control, though working hard, and are not asking for pain relief, you will probably not be offered any. If, on the other hand, you are completely out of control and thrashing about, you may be prolonging your labor, and your caregiver will probably suggest some sort of medication to get you back in control.

14.

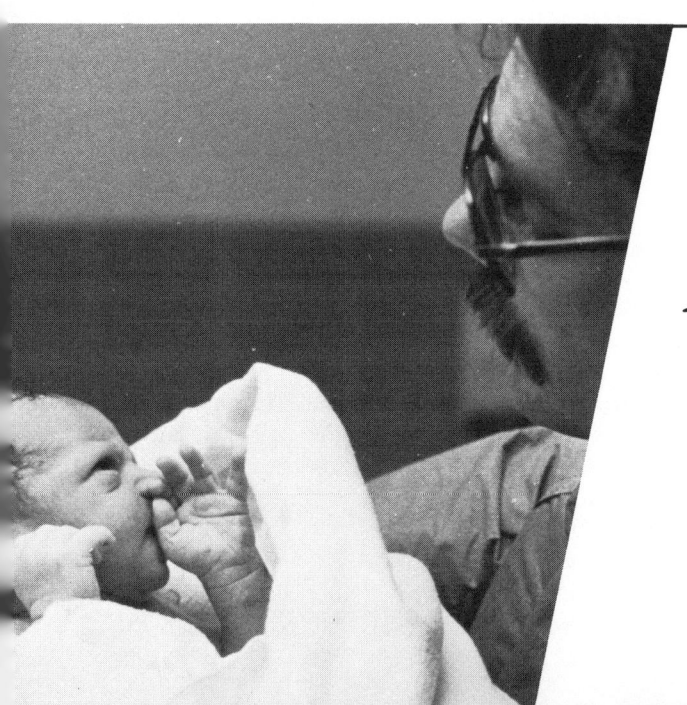

Being Prepared for All Eventualities

How do you know if you are really in active labor? When do you call your husband? When do you call your doctor? When do you go to the hospital? All of these are questions that most women feel unsure about. Everyone wants definite guidelines, but labor starts so differently for each woman that we can only give you some idea of how to judge for yourself. You should definitely call the doctor if you experience any pain, bleeding, or rupture of membranes.

The most reliable sign of active labor is the increasing length, strength, and intensity of the contractions as well as their quality and location. Contractions during active labor usually (but not always) develop a regular pattern and do not go away. They get closer together, stronger, and longer. Your abdomen will feel very hard during a contraction, and you will feel most of the intensity in your back, groin, or above your pubic arch. Walking increases their intensity. A hot bath, heat, alcohol, or sedatives will not stop them.

The contractions of prelabor are just the opposite. They are often irregular, their strength and intensity vary, and they do not establish a pattern. They do not get stronger. If you take a sleeping pill or a glass of wine, the contractions will stop eventually. When you become active or change position, the contractions may stop.

If you think you are in labor, but are not sure, take a little time to analyze your contractions. If you are still uncertain, visit your doctor's office for a quick vaginal check to put your mind at ease. Some hospitals will allow you to come in for a check without first registering.

What do you do if you panic on the way to the hospital? Many times the disruption of the trip from home to the hospital causes a woman to begin to panic. If the coach sees that she is becoming tense, he should have her concentrate on her slow breathing and relaxation as he is driving. Should this not work, the coach should stop the car and begin actively to coach her and stroke her body until he can get her under control to continue the journey.

What do you do if you begin to have the desire to push in the car? Very few coaches want to deliver a baby in the car; on the other hand, every coach worries about it. If this should happen to you, first try to have the woman pant through her contractions; this

TRUE AND FALSE LABOR

	ACTIVE (TRUE) LABOR	EARLY (FALSE) LABOR
PHYSICAL SYMPTOMS	Flulike feeling; sometimes intestinal upset; frequent bowel movements; bloody show may be present; backache	None; no bloody show; may or may not have backache
CONTRACTIONS	*Length:* become increasingly longer *Strength:* become increasingly stronger *Duration:* become increasingly closer *Timing:* Rarely exceed 60 seconds *Place:* Often felt in back, radiating to abdomen *Pattern:* may become increasingly regular	*Length:* varies *Strength:* decreases, and stops *Duration:* varies and stops *Timing:* may last 3–4 minutes *Place:* usually felt in lower part of abdomen and groin *Pattern:* often irregular
MATERNAL ACTIVITY	Walking may increase contractions (they will not subside when she stops walking); hot bath will not stop contractions; alcoholic drink will not stop contractions; changing positions will not stop contractions	Walking: contractions will subside as the mother becomes more (or less) active; activity affects contractions; hot bath will stop contractions; alcohol will stop contractions; changing positions may stop contractions
VAGINAL SIGNS	Heavy discharge; mucus streaked with blood; bloody show	Heavy discharge; little or no bloody show
CERVICAL SIGNS	Cervix is effacing or thinning in a continual pattern of progress; dilatation increases progressively; membranes may be under tension	When checked by examiner, cervix may be effacing, but no showable progress; dilatation: some, but no showable progress; membranes do not feel tense
FETAL ACTIVITY	Baby descends into pelvis (engages with first baby)	No further descent of baby into pelvis

may help counteract the desire to push. If this does not work, stop the car and prepare to deliver your baby (see pages 163–164).

What do you do if you get to the hospital and you find you are only one centimeter dilated? Getting to the hospital too early can precipitate a long and arduous labor, so it is to your advantage to leave the hospital (if you can) and return at a later time. If you are simply in early labor and your membranes have not ruptured, if you have no history of medical or obstetrical problems, and if you live not too far from the hospital, your birthing attendant will probably suggest that you go home. If no one suggests it, you yourself should bring it up. If they do not want you to go home, suggest that you take a long walk outside the hospital, go for a drive, and try to pass the time in an activity that will take your mind off the contractions, but not tire you for the labor that is certainly imminent.

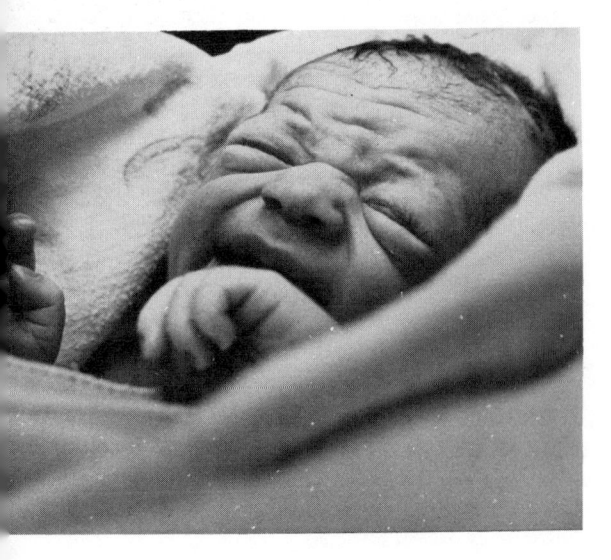

What do you do if your membranes break at home? If, at any time, your membranes rupture, you must call your medical caregiver and let him or her ascertain whether you should come in for care. The usual suggestion is that you wait twenty to twenty-four hours to see if labor begins on its own. If it does not, because there is a possibility of infection, you will probably be told to go to the hospital so that labor may be artificially induced.

What do you do if your coach can't be reached? If you cannot reach your coach, you must call a back-up person. If that person has not been trained you may have to experience labor on your own. Although admittedly more difficult, it is possible, and you must remind yourself that you have the skills and can concentrate on your breathing and relaxation techniques.

What do you do if your nurse asks you why you are doing that crazy breathing? If you happen to get an attendant who does not know about prepared childbirth, you may be asked about your breathing patterns. First, remember that your labor nurse is usually the most important person involved in your labor. She has true concern and has a great deal of experience to help you. Tell her that you have received special preparation for this birth and that birthing patterns are one of the techniques learned that will help you. Suggest that she see if the breathing is a help to you—and that if it doesn't work you would be glad to have any other suggestions from her—but that you do want to try what you have learned. If you are already in intense labor, your coach should explain to the nurse.

What do you do if your nurse asks you if you want anesthetics now? Your problem at this time is to assess three things: how far along you are in labor, how long it took you to get there, and how fast you seem to be moving now. Ask the nurse to check your dilatation. Compare that information with how long it took you to get there. Then ask to be checked later to see how fast you are progressing. For example, if you came into the hospital at 3 P.M. at 3 cm. dilatation, and 4 P.M. your dilatation was 5 cm. and at 5 P.M. it was 6 cm. dilatation, you are moving right along. It would seem that in transition you would move along even more rapidly and that an anesthetic would not be needed. On the other hand, if the nurse checked you at 7 P.M. and you were 7 cm. dilated and at 9 P.M. your cervix was only 7.5 cm. dilated, you might consider some anesthetic to calm you and to relax the cervix to make the contractions more effective.

What do you, the coach, do if you are asked to leave the room? If the safety of the mother or baby is at stake, the greatest favor you can do for yourself, the mother, and the baby is to step out and let the medical team handle the emergency. When there is fetal distress, time is of the essence, and any way that you can help expedite emergency care is important.

If there is no emergency, you have to weigh several factors. First, did you make an agreement with the doctor during prenatal visits that you would be a part of the team? If you did, you need only have the attendant call the doctor; or you yourself may do so. If you had no previous agreement, the labor room is a poor battlefield. Try to understand the attendant's point of view. Explain to him or her the time and effort you have put into preparation for this experience. Try to negotiate some middle ground where you can both come out winning.

What if you give birth on the way to the hospital? We all dream of it, in an unbelieving sort of way. What if we don't make it to the hospital? What if I have to deliver the baby? Well, it probably won't happen to you. But if it does, be prepared.

First, it is nice to know that such spontaneous births are usually very normal, safe, and easy. Second, remember that women have delivered babies for thousands of years without the help of obstetricians, and the coach's role in the birth will probably be minimal. In fact, the less you do to the mother and the baby, the safer it generally will be.

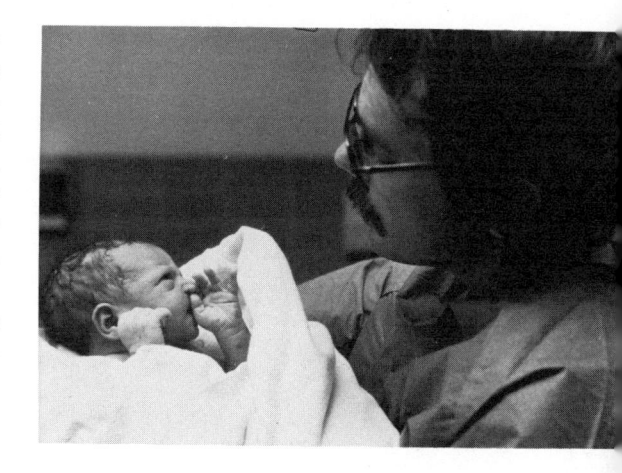

However, there are several things you should keep in mind. First, if the mother begins bearing down and you are in transit in a car, it is probably best that you prepare her a place that is as comfortable and hygienic as possible. The mother's vaginal area must be kept clean. Unopened, clean newspaper is probably as sterile a material as you can find. Open up the newspapers and spread them around the back seat. Remove her panties. Get her in as comfortable a position as you can. As she begins pushing, instruct her to take a breath and bear down slowly and in control. She may be in even more control if, as she is pushing, she slowly lets a stream of air out of her pursed lips. When the baby's head crowns it is important that you command the mother to open her mouth and begin panting, so that the baby slides out slowly and does not tear the mother's perineum. Do not touch the vaginal area.

When the baby's head emerges, instruct the mother to reach down, hold his head, and give another push. When the baby's body is born, place him in a warm clean blanket or shirt with skin-to-skin contact on the mother's breast. Your concern is keeping the baby warm, and the mother's body heat is the best warmth for him. The next part of the birth is delivery of the placenta. The cord is still attached to the baby and to the placenta within the mother's body. Do not touch the cord or pull on it, and do not touch the mother's pelvic floor. The moment the baby is born, the placenta starts to detach itself from the wall of the uterus. With the next contraction (or contractions), the placenta will be expelled on its own. Wrap it in newspaper and place it alongside the baby and mother with the cord still attached to the baby. Do not cut the cord. You usually do not have to worry about the baby breathing because such spontaneous and short births tend to deliver very alert babies who cry right away.

Now, your third and last concern: the mother's bleeding from the uterine site where the placenta detached itself. If you let nature take its own way, you can control even this. When you put the baby to the mother's breast, its licking and sucking causes the uterine muscles to clamp down on the placental site and stop the bleeding.

Now, all you must do is keep the mother and baby warm, and get them to a place where the umbilical cord can be cut and the placenta checked to see that all parts were delivered and nothing left inside the mother.

And, once you have been through all this, you will have a story to tell for many years.

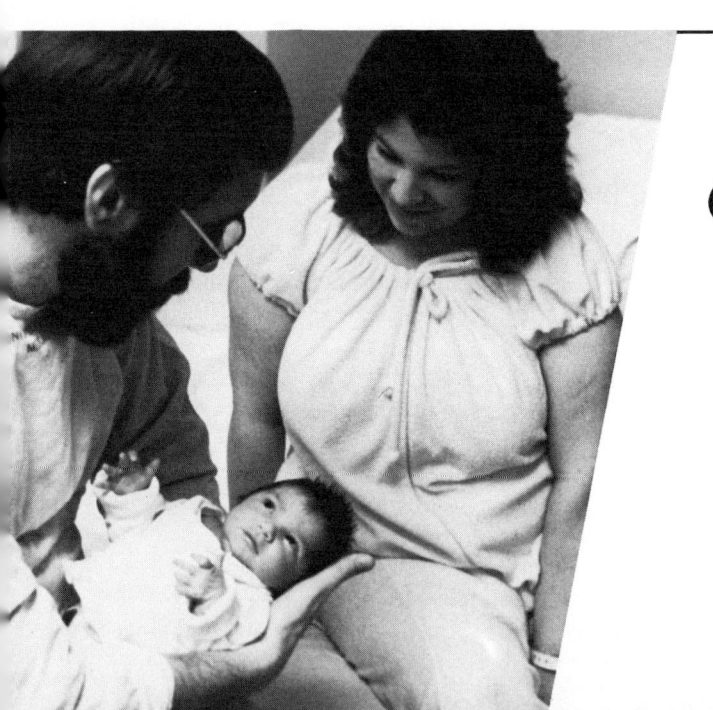

Glossary

Afterbirth: The placenta and membranes that are expelled after the birth of the baby.

Afterpains: Uterine cramping caused by contractions of the uterus following birth.

Amniocentesis: A medical procedure involving the withdrawal of amniotic fluid from a pregnant woman for the purpose of evaluating the fetus.

Amniotic fluid: An amber-colored liquid filling the uterus of a pregnant woman that cushions the baby from injury and maintains a constant temperature.

Amniotic sac: A sac of thin membranes that surround the baby and the amniotic fluid in a pregnant woman; commonly called the "bag of waters."

Amniotomy: A medical procedure that artificially ruptures the membranes to induce labor.

Analgesic: A drug that lessens the perception of pain.

Anesthetic: General: A drug that produces total loss of consciousness; given intravenously or inhaled. *Local:* A drug that diminishes or eliminates sensation from a specific body part. Examples include the paracervical block, the pudendal block, and local infiltration of the perineum.

Anesthesiologist: A physician whose specialty is administering local and general anesthetics.

Anesthetist: A nurse trained to monitor a patient after the anesthesia has been administered.

Anus: The external opening of the rectum.

Apgar score: A score derived from evaluating a newborn one minute and five minutes after birth. Heart rate, respiratory effort, muscle tone, reflexes, and the color of the baby are all factors in the evaluation.

Bag of waters: See *Amniotic sac.*

Birth canal: The bony passageway of the mother's pelvis and the vagina through which a baby passes during birth.

Blood pressure: Tension produced by the blood current on the walls of the blood vessels.

Bloody show: Blood-tinged mucus expelled by a pregnant woman prior to labor. This indicates a softening of the cervix and the release of the mucous plug.

Bradycardia: A slow heart rate in an infant; measured by a fetal monitor during labor to indicate an infant's response to the stress of contractions.

Braxton-Hicks contractions: Uterine contractions occurring periodically throughout pregnancy. Toward the end of pregnancy they may become more persistent and uncomfortable and be difficult to discern from early or active labor—thus the term, "false labor."

Breech: The baby's presentation in labor in which the buttocks, rather than the head, are situated at the cervix.

Catheterization: The continual emptying of the bladder by the insertion of a small tube through the urethra into the bladder.

Centimeter: A metric unit of measurement used to measure cervical dilatation. One inch equals about 2.5 centimeters; complete dilatation is 10 centimeters (or about four inches).

Cephalopelvic disproportion (CPD): A mismatch between the size of the mother's pelvis and the size of the baby's head.

Cervix: The neck of the uterus—the passageway from the uterus to the vagina.

Cesarean section (C-section): Birth in which the baby is delivered through a surgical incision in the abdominal wall and the uterus.

Coccyx: The small bone at the end of the spinal column beyond the sacrum. Commonly called the "tailbone."

Clitoris: Located above the urinary opening, the clitoris is the female organ of sexual pleasure.

Colostrum: The first substance produced by the milk glands. A thick sticky yellow fluid high in proteins and antibodies that is the forerunner of milk.

Contraction: The tightening and shortening of a muscle. Uterine contractions occur during labor and they change in length, frequency, and intensity. *Length* is the time from the beginning of the contraction to the end of the contraction. *Frequency* is the time elapsing from the beginning of one contraction to the beginning of the next contraction. *Intensity* is the strength of the contraction.

Cord: See *Umbilical cord.*

Crowning: The appearance of the largest part of the baby's head at the vaginal outlet during the expulsion.

Dilatation: The opening of the cervix during labor from 0 cm. to 10 cm. (complete dilatation).

Dystocia: A condition in which the cervix fails to dilate effectively during labor.

Effacement: The thinning and shortening of the cervix into the body of the uterus. It may occur prior to or simultaneously with dilatation prior to childbirth.

Effleurage: A light stroking massage over the abdomen during labor.

Engagement: The descent of the baby's presenting part into the pelvis to zero station (or to the level of the ischial spines).

Episiotomy: An incision made at the vaginal outlet from the vagina toward the anus.

Estimated due date (EDD or EDC): Estimated date of confinement.

Expulsion: The pushing efforts of the mother combined with the force of the uterine contractions, resulting in the delivery of the baby.

False labor: Recurring contractions that may seem like labor, but do not dilate the cervix (see *Braxton-Hicks contractions*). Now called prelabor, these contractions are preparing the uterus for actual labor.

Fetal distress: Physical stress of the infant in the uterus, caused by conditions of the uterine environment or contractions during labor. Fetal distress is signaled by a slowing down or speeding up of the baby's heart tones, or by meconium staining in the amniotic fluid.

Fetal heart tones (FHT): The fetus's, or baby's, heart tones, which average about 140 beats per minute (or between 120 and 160).

Fetal monitor: An electronic machine used to detect and record fetal heart tones and their reactions to the stresses of the contractions of labor. It may be attached internally through the vagina or externally over the mother's abdomen.

Fetus: The developing baby from three months until birth.

Forceps: An obstetrical instrument used to assist in delivery of the baby.

Fundus: The uppermost portion of the uterus that lies above the fallopian tubes and expands the greatest amount in order to allow for the growth of the fetus.

Gravida: The state of being pregnant; the number of times a woman has been pregnant. Primigravida indicates a first pregnancy; multigravida indicates that pregnancy has occurred more than once.

Hyperventilation: An imbalance of oxygen and carbon dioxide in the body caused by breathing that is too deep or too fast. Symptoms are dizziness, light-headedness, and tingling or numbness around the lips, fingers, and toes.

Induction: Labor started by artificial methods, usually by either rupturing the membranes or by the administration of the hormone pitocin.

Intravenous infusion (IV): Administration of fluids through the vein for the purposes of nutrition, hydration, or medication.

Labia: The external folds around the opening of the vagina.

Labor: The process by which periodic and rhythmic contractions efface and dilate the cervix prior to delivery.

Lamaze method: The Lamaze method, or the psychoprophylactic method (PPM) of childbirth is based on the laboring woman using her brain to interpret and respond to her contractions with relaxation, breathing, massage, and focal point techniques to prevent or alleviate painful sensations.

Lightening: The lowered level of the uterus that results from the baby dropping into the pelvic inlet during engagement. Commonly called "dropping."

Membranes: See *Amniotic sac.*

Midwife: Nurse midwives are professionally educated and trained to manage a normal labor and delivery and to recognize complications and refer them to physicians for treatment. Lay midwives have usually experienced birth firsthand and wish to share their knowledge with other mothers.

Molding: The shaping of the baby's head during childbirth to adapt to the size and contours of the mother's pelvis and birth canal.

Mucous plug: The mucus that blocks the cervical canal of a woman during pregnancy to prevent the entry of germs into the uterus.

Multigravida: See *Gravida.*

Obstetrician: A physician specializing in the care of pregnant women and in the delivery of babies.

Occiput: A term referring to the back of the head.

Oxytocin: A hormone secreted by the pituitary gland that influences the uterus to contract.

Pelvic floor: A muscular sling that supports the rectum, urethra, bladder, and internal reproductive organs.

Pelvis: The bony basin formed by the sacrum, coccyx, and hip bones.

Perineum: The tissue surrounding the area between the vagina and the anus.

Pitocin: A synthetic hormone used to induce uterine contractions.

Phases of labor: A term used to describe the physical and emotional characteristics of the early, active, and transitional phases a woman passes through in labor.

Placenta: A spongelike organ that provides nourishment and oxygen and eliminates waste products for the fetus during pregnancy.

Position: The relationship of the presenting part of the baby to the front, back, or sides of the woman's pelvis (anterior, posterior).

Posterior position: A position of the baby in which the back of the baby's head (occiput) lies toward the back of the woman's pelvis.

Postmature: A baby who is born after 42 weeks of gestation in the uterus.

Postpartum: The period of time after birth.

Precipitous labor: A labor and delivery that is extremely rapid, involving less than three hours' total time.

Premature: A term used to describe a baby born with a weight of less than 5 pounds, 8 ounces, or a baby that is born before 40 weeks' gestation.

Prep: A hospital procedure in which a laboring woman is given an enema, a partial shave of the pubic hair, blood tests, and a physical examination. A medical history is taken at this time.

Presentation: A term used to refer to the part of the baby lying nearest the cervix: cephalic (head), breech (buttocks), or shoulder.

Primigravida: See *Gravida*.

Prolapsed cord: An umbilical cord that is expelled before the presenting part of the baby.

Psychoprophylaxis: See *Lamaze method*.

Pubic symphysis: The area joining the two bones in front of the pelvis. This joint softens during pregnancy.

Rectum: The lower part of the intestine leading to the anal opening.

Ripening: A softening of the cervical tissues caused by hormones released during the latter part of pregnancy.

Rupture of membranes: The rupture of the amniotic membranes, occurring spontaneously before or during labor. The membranes may also be ruptured artificially by the birthing attendant to bring on labor.

Sacrum: The lower triangular bone that connects the spinal column to the pelvis.

Show: The expulsion of the mucous plug combined with slight bleeding is commonly called "bloody show."

Spinal: An anesthetic introduced into the spinal area to numb the body from the breasts to the feet.

Stages of birth: The division of the entire physiological birth process: first stage: labor; second stage: delivery; third stage: expulsion of the placenta; fourth stage: immediate postpartum.

Station: A measurement of the progress of the baby's descent in the mother's pelvis.

Stripping of the membranes: A process whereby the birthing attendant inserts a finger into the vagina and separates the amniotic sac from the cervix to induce labor.

Term: The complete cycle of pregnancy at 38–42 weeks' gestation.

Tranquilizer: Medication that relieves apprehension and gives a feeling of calmness.

Transition: The third phase of labor in which the cervix is dilated from 7–10 cm. and the mother begins to feel the urge to push.

True labor: Uterine contractions that affect continual progressive effacement and dilatation of the cervix.

Ultrasound: A device using high-frequency sound waves to locate the placenta and to obtain measurements of the baby's head and chest, used to determine the gestational age of the fetus.

Umbilical cord: The tubelike structure 12–20 inches in length connecting the placenta to the baby. The umbilical cord contains two arteries and one vein that carry nutrients and oxygen to the baby and eliminate waste products.

Umbilicus: The area where the umbilical cord was attached to the uterus. Commonly called the "belly button," or "navel."

Uterine inertia: Contractions during labor which are short, weak, infrequent and/or erratic and are not effective in dilating the cervix.

Uterus: The female organ that receives the fertilized egg, supports and nurtures it during pregnancy, and contracts during expulsion.

Vagina: The female birth canal and the organ for sexual intercourse.

Vertex (cephalic): A term used to indicate that the part of the baby presenting itself to the cervix is the head.

Vital signs: Signs that show the body's response to life processes, including respiration, pulse, and temperature.

Vulva: The external female anatomy, which includes the labia majora, labia minora, and clitoris.

Womb: See *Uterus*.

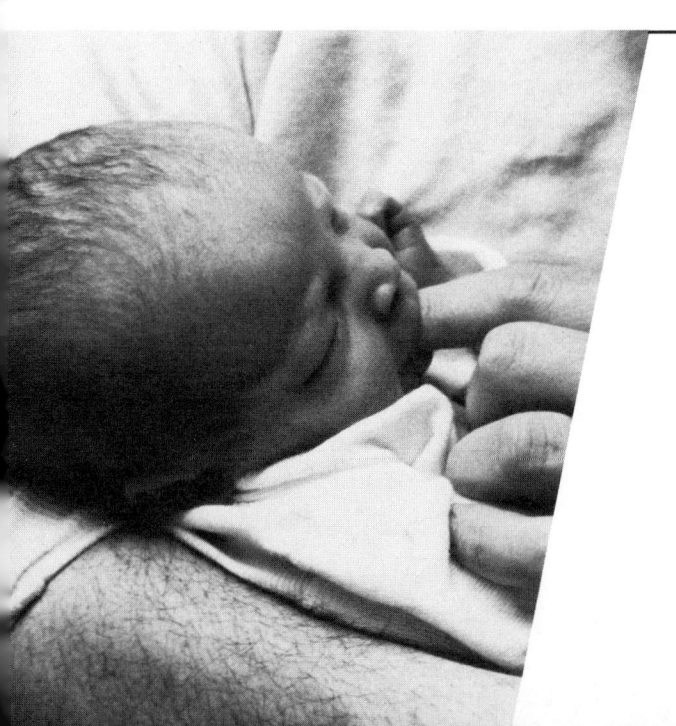

Further Reading

The Boston Women's Health Collective. *Our Bodies, Ourselves.* New York: Simon & Schuster, 1976.

CHABON, IRWIN. *Awake and Aware: Participating in Childbirth Through Psychoprophylaxis.* New York: Delacorte, 1966.

CLARK, ANN L. et al. *Childbearing: A Nursing Perspective.* Philadelphia: F. A. Davis Co., 1979.

CLAUSEN, JOY et al. *Maternity Nursing Today.* New York: McGraw-Hill, 1976.

DONOVAN, BONNIE. *The Cesarean Birth Experience: A Practical, Comprehensive, and Reassuring Guide for Parents and Professionals.* Boston: Beacon Press, 1977.

EWY, DONNA, and RODGER EWY. *Preparation for Childbirth: A Lamaze Guide.* New York: Signet Books, 1970.

GARREY, MATTHEW M. et al. *Obstetrics Illustrated.* New York: Churchill Livingstone Inc., 1980.

HAUSKNECHT, RICHARD, and JOAN R. HEILMAN. *Having a Cesarean Baby.* New York: E. P. Dutton, 1978.

KARMEL, MAJORIE. *Thank You, Dr. Lamaze.* New York: Harper & Row, 1981.

KITZINGER, SHEILA. *Giving Birth: The Patients' Emotions in Childbirth.* New York: Taplinger, 1971.

KLAUS, MARSHALL, and JOHN KENNELL. *Maternal-Infant Bonding.* St. Louis, Missouri: Mosby Press, 1976.

LAMAZE, FERNAND. *Painless Childbirth.* New York: Pocket Books, 1977.

LEBOYER, FREDERICK. *Birth Without Violence.* New York: Alfred A. Knopf, 1975.

MACFARLANE, AIDAN. *The Psychology of Childbirth.* Cambridge, Massachusetts: Harvard University Press, 1977.

MYLES, MARGARET. *A Textbook for Midwives.* New York: Churchill Livingstone Inc., 1975.

OXORN. *Human Labor and Birth.* New York: Appleton-Century-Crofts, 1975.

REEDER, SHARON R. et al. *Maternity Nursing.* New York: J. B. Lippincott, 1980.

TANZER, DEBORAH, and JEAN L. BLOCK. *Why Natural Childbirth? A Psychologist's Report on the Benefits to Mothers, Fathers, and Babies.* New York: Schocken Books, 1976.

WALTON, VICKIE. *Have It Your Way.* New York: Bantam Books, 1976.

WESSEL, HELEN. *The Joy of Natural Childbirth.* New York: Harper & Row, 1976.